Mastering Mentorship

A Practical Guide for Mentors
of Nursing, Health and Social Care Students

ulie Bailey-McHale and Donna Hart

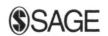

Los Angeles | London | New Delhi
Singapore | Washington DC

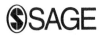

Los Angeles | London | New Delhi
Singapore | Washington DC

SAGE Publications Ltd
1 Oliver's Yard
55 City Road
London EC1Y 1SP

SAGE Publications Inc.
2455 Teller Road
Thousand Oaks, California 91320

SAGE Publications India Pvt Ltd
B 1/I 1 Mohan Cooperative Industrial Area
Mathura Road
New Delhi 110 044

SAGE Publications Asia-Pacific Pte Ltd
3 Church Street
#10-04 Samsung Hub
Singapore 049483

Editor: Alex Clabburn
Assistant editor: Emma Milman
Production editor: Katie Forsythe
Copyeditor: Audrey Scriven
Proofreader: Neil Dowden
Marketing manager: Tamara Navaratnam
Cover design: Naomi Robinson
Typeset by: C&M Digitals (P) Ltd, Chennai, India
Printed and bound by MPG Printgroup, UK

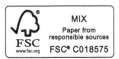

First published 2013

Library of Congress Control Number: 2012949940

British Library Cataloguing in Publication data

A catalogue record for this book is available from the British
Library

ISBN 978-0-85702-982-9
ISBN 978-0-85702-983-6 (pbk)

Mastering
Mentorship

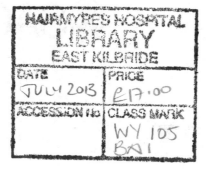

SAGE has been part of the global academic community since 1965, supporting high quality research and learning that transforms society and our understanding of individuals, groups and cultures. SAGE is the independent, innovative, natural home for authors, editors and societies who share our commitment and passion for the social sciences.

Find out more at: **www.sagepublications.com**

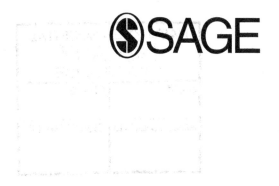

For Mike McHale (1936–2011), who gave his daughters the most precious of gifts – the courage to dare to dream. This is for you, Dad!

For David 'Tim' Hart (1941–1991), who is so proud of every little thing my sister and I achieve.

Contents

About the Authors

Julie Bailey-McHale is a Senior Lecturer in the Health and Social Care Teaching Team, Department of Health, Isle of Man. She is programme leader for the pre-registration mental health nursing programme and leads a number of modules at levels 6 and 7 on both mental health and mentorship. She qualified as a mental health nurse in 1990 and has worked in acute inpatient and forensic settings. She moved into nurse education in 2002 and worked at the University of Chester where she developed an interest in mentorship and has pursued this interest with enthusiasm on her move to the Isle of Man. She has developed strong collaborative links across mental health services. She is currently studying for a PhD.

Donna Hart is a Principal Lecturer in the Health and Social Care Teaching Team, Department of Health, Isle of Man. She has responsibilities for pre- and post-registration programmes and leads on a number of modules at levels 6 and 7 including public health and mentorship. She has enjoyed a career in nursing, qualifying in 1986, initially working in a surgical area before moving into the community in 1988, and qualifying as a District Nurse in 1990. She moved into nurse education in 1995 and worked at the University of Brighton as a Senior Lecturer in Community Nursing. On moving to the Isle of Man in 2000 she built on an existing interest in mentorship and has contributed to the strategic development of mentorship on the Isle of Man.

Foreword

Susan Bernhauser

I was delighted to be invited to write the Foreword for this book, which is a long overdue text linking the theoretical underpinnings of mentorship to the art and practice of it.

It recognises the pivotal role of mentorship within the experience of health and social care students, whatever their level of study, and is particularly timely with the move of nursing to an all graduate profession at the point of registration.

As a University Dean with exposure to students from the health, social care and other practice-based disciplines there is evidence, and anecdote, that confirms the importance of mentors in moulding and modelling the development of safe, competent practitioners and to support the development of appropriate attitudes and behaviours which underpin professional practice.

Reports such as those produced by the recent Commission on Nurse Education, chaired by Lord Willis of Knaresborough (Royal College of Nursing, November 2012), the Prime Minister's Commission on the Future of Nursing and Midwifery (Prime Minister's Office, March 2010) and numerous reports from professional and statutory bodies all provide evidence of the importance of high quality, well-informed mentorship for students in practice. Students, in giving evidence to these commissions, said that good mentorship was the one thing that 'made a real difference'.

This book deals with the traditional thorny issues surrounding the compatibility, or not, of the mentor assessing student practice. The multifaceted role of the mentor is explored with the use of case studies and bravely recognises the inherent contradictions within some of those roles.

It takes the reader through the support and key leadership needed in mentorship from organisational level through to the individual mentor and mentee. Identifying the fundamental importance of positive and productive relationships that are needed between health care providers and universities, the mentor is found at the forefront and operational end of that relationship; the cement that binds it together.

The case studies within the book carefully illuminate important issues in a pragmatic way, offering, in many cases, helpful strategies and insights to enhance mentorship for both the mentor and mentee. The learning objectives at the end of each chapter serve to ask the reader to reflect on the content and undertake activities which develop understanding and learning.

This book deals with the 'how' and 'what' of mentorship, as well as the context in which it is delivered. With the careful use of real world examples and exemplars it recognises the reality of balancing mentorship with the delivery of care and services to patients and clients. It offers teaching opportunities for mentor preparation and the opportunity to explore it's theoretical basis.

Although the chapters could stand alone, they provide a rich exploration of the role of the mentor and offer insights into its complexity. The book explores the situations and challenges inherent in this important role and the many personal, professional and organisational factors which can influence it.

For practitioners undertaking the mentorship role it offers the opportunity to develop areas of potential improvement and revisit some fundamental principles.

This book underpins the Master's level education of those professionals, in practice, who are central in the development of the next generation of health and social care practitioners.

In conclusion this book needs to be in libraries that support health and social care professional education, on the bookshelves and desks of professionals who take this role on, or support it, providing everything from helpful insights to new theoretical perspectives.

Susan Bernhauser
Emerita Dean of Human and Health Sciences,
University of Huddersfield

Previous Chair of the Council of Deans of Health UK

Acknowledgements

We would like to thank the following people for their help and support throughout the process of writing this book.

Our gratitude must go to Pauline Golding for her patience and humour through hours of proofreading and formatting. Also to our colleagues at Keyll Darree for putting up with our occasional states of distraction and helping in ways too numerous to list.

We send heartfelt thanks to our families, Michael, Emily, Josh, Lisa, Ron and Len, and to our mums. Special thanks goes to Bex for all the love, support and patience throughout.

Finally, to all the case study authors – thank you for your continued support of learners and for bringing to life and sharing your experiences of mentorship within your case study contributions.

Introduction

The old adage of George Bernard Shaw suggesting those who can, do, and those who can't, teach, is undoubtedly challenged by the role of the mentor in professional practice. Mentors in health and social care practice must not only 'do the do' but must also be able to teach that 'do'. Mentors along with colleagues in practice and the wider learning organisation require passion and enthusiasm for mentorship. They also need to value and have a belief in the merits of mentorship and an understanding of the evidence to underpin this fundamental role. We hope to demonstrate these qualities throughout this book. In it we will explore the complexity of the role of mentor, preceptor and supervisor, as well as celebrate the mastery required to perform this role well. At its heart is the desire to demonstrate that mentors utilise Master's level thinking skills in the advanced practice activity of mentoring in professional education. As health and social care professions negotiate their way through the second decade of this century they will continue to look for innovative and effective ways to teach the art of their professional practice.

The move to a degree-only preparation for nursing, the inclusion of social work within the Health and Care Profession's Council and increasing political and economic uncertainty have all contributed to a growing scrutiny of pre-qualifying professional programmes. The continuing professional development of qualified health and social care practitioners is also under examination. The 'appalling suffering of many patients' detailed in the Francis Report (2013: 3) highlights in stark terms the multitude of failings within the healthcare system. The role of mentors in supporting health and social care students to develop the professional curiosity and courage to always put their patients first is now more crucial than ever.

This book will define, contextualise and present theoretical explanations of mentorship and we hope its chapters will demonstrate both the art and craft of mentorship, supervision and preceptorship. We believe their content will resonate across health and social care professions and will also have value for health and social care practice education colleagues internationally. A unique feature of the book is the inclusion throughout of contributions by Master's level health and social care student mentors, who showcase the complexity of the integration of the theory and practice of effective mentoring. The chapters are divided using the Nursing and Midwifery Council (2008) domains described in the Standards to Support Learning and Assessment in Practice (NMC, 2008). These domains are establishing effective working relationships, the facilitation of learning, assessment and accountability, evaluation, creating an environment for learning, the context of practice, evidence-based practice and leadership. Although nursing led, these reflect the various skills, knowledge and values that are required to mentor regardless of the health and social care professional role and are widely acknowledged within professional practice education literature. These domains are implicit within the Health and Care Professions Council Standards for Education and Training (HCPC, 2012). In addition, The College of Social Work are in the process of phasing in new practice educator standards for social work (TCSW, 2012). Those standards detail four domains: to organise opportunities for the demonstration of assessed competence in practice; to enable learning and professional development in practice; to manage the assessment of learners in practice; and effective continuing performance as a practice educator. Throughout the book both the HCPC (2012) standards and TCSW (2012) standards will be directly referred to.

Each chapter is supported by a number of case studies which reflect the practical application of the key theoretical features discussed within that chapter. The case studies have been written by health and social care professionals who are currently actively involved in mentorship in its broadest terms. All of the case study contributors have successfully completed a Master's mentorship module delivered by the authors. Indeed it was the quality of this academic work that led the authors to consider writing this book. The case studies showcase key mentorship issues within contemporary health and social care practice and how our mentors, often through innovative approaches, demonstrated their mastery in mentorship.

Chapter 1 explores the current landscape of mentorship and links this to the qualities and knowledge mentors require to do this role well. The authors will demonstrate that the qualities associated with Master's level study and practice are essential to achieving excellence in mentoring. The complexities of mentorship in practice demand higher level thinking skills and particularly require mentors to deal with uncertainty and difficult decisions. The case study within this chapter provides a personal reflection regarding the experience and expertise that are necessary to mentor and links these to the academic level of study.

Chapter 2 discusses the nature of relationships within mentoring and the importance of an effective relationship between the mentor and mentee. The skill of facilitating effective learning in practice and assessing such learning appropriately ultimately relies on the strength of that relationship. In the chapter three case studies are used to show the complexities of the mentoring relationship. The first of these reviews the use of a coaching model within a social work mentorship relationship and describes the ways in which the case study author has successfully implemented this approach with postgraduate social work students. The second case study takes the reader to the operating theatre and explores the effect of assessment on the mentorship relationship. The case study author here explores the skills required to unpick the delicate balance between mentor and assessor within the context of an effective relationship. The third case study author is a nurse in an accident and emergency department and demonstrates the important characteristics required within the mentor/mentee relationship.

A key feature of the mentoring role is the effective and creative facilitation and structuring of the learning experience. Chapter 3 explores the ways in which learning can be facilitated across a range of health and social care settings. It offers practical examples of the integration of learning theories to ensure the effective facilitation of learning. There are four case studies presented within this chapter. Two of the case study authors look at reflection as a means of facilitating learning: the first case study explores the difficulties associated with moving from the role of expert to novice within professional practice (examining the strategies used within a Children's Centre to assist staff in this transition and to build confidence and expertise within a new set of skills); the second looks at the application of key learning theories to the facilitation of learning in practice (using a district nursing setting). The third case study describes an innovative Practice Guide role (created within a pre-registration mental health nursing programme). A key feature of the Practice Guide role is to undertake structured, facilitated clinical supervision sessions with student mental health nurses in order to facilitate the linking of mental health nursing theory and practice. A final case study examines the merits and challenges of using reflection to facilitate learning in a community-based drug and alcohol team.

Chapter 4 goes on to highlight innovative ways in which practice can be assessed across health and social care and the role and accountability of the mentor within the assessment process. The three case studies within this chapter take a wide-ranging view of assessment. The first case study highlights the merits of reflection within the assessment process: it is set within a health visiting team and explores the ways in which reflection can be used to aid assessment. The second case study author describes some of the issues involved in assessing the ongoing competence of registered professionals. The final case study considers the use of service user feedback to inform the personal and professional development plans of staff: the author looks at the challenges of doing this in a district nursing practice setting.

Chapter 5 details the importance of the evaluation of the learning experience and the various methods used to evaluate learning in practice. Evaluation is embedded in the quality processes of both practice and academic institutions, and in the case study for this chapter the author will address some of the inconsistencies for nurse mentors in evaluating their own mentorship practice.

The impact of the learning environment on the mentee's learning is explored in Chapter 6, in particular the need for mentors to organise the environment to ensure it is conducive to learning. The concept of the learning organisation is also reviewed within this chapter. The three case studies presented reflect a range of themes connected to the learning environment. The first of these takes the theme of reflection and considers whether reflective practice can enhance the learning environment within a health visiting team. The next two case studies explore the importance of the practice learning environment in pre-registration nursing: the first is within a school nursing team and the second is situated within a multi-professional community mental health team. Both look at the appropriateness of the learning environment for the student nurses allocated to their respective teams.

Chapter 7 reviews the various practice contexts in which learning takes place and examines especially the ways in which learning happens in practice and the potential barriers to this learning. The first case study highlights some of the tensions and challenges faced by the mentor when supporting a reluctant learner. The second considers the skills involved in health promotion and relates these skills to those of a mentor, with the similarities between the two roles also being discussed. The third case study explores the impact of inter-professional working and learning within a multi-professional community drug and alcohol team and the ways in which a social work student can engage fully in this learning environment. Finally, the challenge of transforming 'ordinary' practice situations into a meaningful learning opportunity is considered. The author in this fourth case study describes how the daily morning meeting in a Children's Centre has incorporated a reflective approach to encourage critical reflection within the team.

Chapter 8 examines the role of evidence-based health and social care and the implications of this for practice mentors. It also explores the notion of values-based practice and the ways in which both evidence- and values-based practice are essential for the development of health and social care students. The case study in this chapter considers the barriers to learning in relation to continuing professional development and the ability to engage in evidence-based practice.

Chapter 9 explores the nature of leadership within health and social care practice and professional education. It examines the skills required by mentors to lead both practice and practice education. The first case study within this chapter describes the challenges inherent in being the leader of a team, a manager and a mentor. The second case study considers the most appropriate leadership style for mentorship.

The final chapter draws together key learning from the previous chapters and discusses the future of mentorship within health and social care professions. The case study is written by the two authors of this book and describes their successful efforts to deliver mentor preparation modules at academic levels six and seven only. The rationale for this is explored and the implications for the future delivery of mentor preparation programmes are examined.

The reader is encouraged to use the Chapter Link boxes found throughout the chapters to review their current understanding of each topic. These Chapter Links act as signposts by indicating the key chapters which discuss a topic further. Each chapter ends with a series of questions to help the reader in applying the contents of that chapter to their own practice setting. The reader is encouraged to use this checklist to consolidate their learning and also to begin to apply it to their own practice as a mentor.

References

Francis, R. (2013) *Report of the Mid-Staffordshire NHS Foundation Trust Public Enquiry. Executive Summary.* London: HMSO.

Health and Care Professions Council (2012) *Standards of Education and Training.* London: HCPC.

Nursing and Midwifery Council (2008) *Standards to Support Learning and Assessment in Practice.* London: NMC.

The College of Social Work (2012) *Practice Educator Professional Standards for Social Work.* London: TCSW.

1   Mastery and Mentorship

Case study: Lisa Hall

There has been widespread recognition for some time of the value of a Master's level qualification for advanced or specialist practitioners within health and social care practice. However, the move to all-graduate preparation for nurses, placing nursing programmes alongside other health and social care pre-qualifying programmes, will inevitably open up the potential for more Master's level pre-qualifying programmes. Clearly this has implications for the preparation of those who mentor health and social care students. This chapter will contextualise mentor preparation within contemporary political, professional and economic drivers. It will offer definitions of mentorship within pre-qualifying professional programmes and define what is involved in the mastery of professional practice. It will then consider these two aspects in conjunction with a discussion of academic descriptions of Master's level study. The chapter will then synthesise the attributes associated with both mentorship and the mastery of professional practice and demonstrate the inherent connectedness of these advanced professional activities to the academic characteristics of Master's level study.

Context

Both professionally and politically there has been a recent focus on the quality of care within health and social care professions. A number of high profile cases across the media have highlighted deficiencies in care provision. These include concerns regarding the standard of nursing for older people and those with learning disabilities and concerns about social work education particularly in relation to safeguarding children. The current economic and political climate has produced unprecedented constraints on health and social care provision and on society as a whole. As with any demographic changes these austerity measures inevitably impact upon the profile of those wishing to enter the health and social care professions. Arguably, factors such as graduate unemployment, redundancies and general job insecurity will increase the number of graduates wishing to enter pre-qualifying programmes. These changes may make those purchasing pre-qualifying professional programmes much more cognisant of the economic sense of providing newly qualified practitioners who are already at Master's level. Most recently the Nursing and Midwifery Council (2010) have revised the standards of education for pre-registration nursing programmes. These now clearly state what is expected of a nurse in contemporary health and social care practice and also more clearly embed Master's level preparation within the pre-registration programme.

These demographic and professional changes inevitably impact on the role and scope of the mentor in professional practice. It seems timely now to raise the profile of mentors to ensure that the value, complexity and centrality of the role is recognised and to consider the advanced nature of mentorship. We would advocate that mentorship is an advanced professional activity and currently effective qualified mentors practise their mentorship at Master's level. Therefore mentorship preparation should move towards that level.

Defining mentorship and mastery in professional practice

There are numerous definitions of mentorship and in much of the literature there is concern regarding the inter-changeable nature of the terms 'mentor', 'supervisor' and 'assessor'. Shardlow (2012) identifies the complexities regarding terminology relating to learning and teaching within social work professional education. He highlights four dimensions to this complexity: these are the current use of a variety of terms such as 'Practice Educator' and 'Practice Assessor'; the inconsistent use of terminology across health and social care disciplines; an international inconsistency in the interpretation and application of terminology; and the fact that all of this is compounded by the theoretical assumptions generated by particular terminology. Whilst the complexities around terminology and theoretical assumptions are a consideration, for over ten years the assessment of competence and fitness to practice has been included within the role of the professional supporting a student on a pre-qualifying programme. It is hoped the following definition clarifies the complexity of the role and is clear about what a mentor does. We would offer the following definition of mentorship which applies to pre-qualifying education programmes. Mentorship is a relationship in which an individual nurtures in another professionally defined values, knowledge and skills which ultimately result in a judgement being made regarding the mentee's competence. This definition describes the mentoring role within pre-qualifying professional programmes; there are, however, a number of different mentorship relationships that are often characterised as being of long duration, informal, mainly formative and mentee selected. It is clear within current professional pre-qualifying programmes where students have to meet defined criteria that these characteristics are not appropriate.

The primary role of a mentor is that of professional practice. We would argue that the skills required and demonstrated within effective mentorship are embedded within the practice of the professional before mentorship preparation is undertaken. Therefore it is important to consider what is Master's level professional practice. Mastery of professional practice can be defined as demonstrating the ability to make sense of complex and divergent concepts, ideas and theories and applying new perspectives in innovative and creative ways with confidence and authority. This mastery within professional practice enables the practitioner to transfer those skills to the activity of mentoring. The following case study is different from others included in the book in that it demonstrates a mentor's personal reflection regarding an aspect of her practice. Lisa Hall considers the appropriate level of experience and knowledge required by a nurse to enable reflection in others and makes reference to the advanced nature of this activity, pulling out some important themes for mentors.

A personal reflection on the level of skill nurses require in order to effectively facilitate reflection in student nurses – Lisa Hall

In my work area mentorship skills are required by registered nurses in order to facilitate learning in student nurses, health care assistants and newly qualified nurses. After one year of being qualified, nurses can become stage two mentors responsible for the formal assessment of

(Continued)

CASE STUDY

(Continued)

students' total performance, facilitating and supervising learning opportunities as well as ensuring standards of proficiency are met (Nursing and Midwifery Council [NMC], 2008). However Neary (2000) agrees with Benner's (1984) suggestion that nurses are only competent to mentor after three years' qualification. Furthermore, after meeting additional criteria mentors can undertake a student's final assessment acting as sign-off mentor (NMC, 2008). To declare a student as 'fit to practice' as a nurse or to fail them requires absolute confidence in and justification of the decision-making process. In a recent *Nursing Times* survey 37 per cent of mentors admitted passing students whom they had concerns about (Gainsbury, 2010). Additionally, Nettleton and Bray (2008) discussed concerns regarding newly qualified nurses' 'fitness to practice' following Project 2000 and as a result of a number of these concerns every student now requires a mentor in the practice setting. With this increased demand, the role can often be imposed upon nurses with the assumption that they have the qualities to mentor and mentoring becomes driven by quantity rather than quality. Arguably this de-values the role and skill of a mentor. With these concerns and the potential impact on the nursing professional and patient care, the role of mentor has never been so vital in ensuring that students proceed onto the register as safe and proficient nurses.

A core aspect of student learning and development is the reflection that mentors facilitate, linking theory to practice by examining an experience, situation or feeling and generating critical thinking and a synthesis of ideas, thereby enhancing knowledge and learning (Moon, 2007). Reflection requires self-awareness and the non-linear thinking that helps to guide decision making and avoids being led by subjective influences. Behaviour that is emulated, which the author terms 'professional hereditary', requires filtration so that students will see 'true' mentoring skills and not just traits acquired from others.

Greenwood (1998) suggests reflection occurs before action necessitating leadership, critical analysis and prioritisation skills and in that action there is the use of clinical judgement, experience and intuition. In addition reflection on action occurs using assessment and synthesis skills, and the seeking of alternatives and changes in perspectives. These skills reflect a level of mastery in mentorship, experience and education and even more so now with nursing moving to all-degree preparation.

Nurses may be perceived to be experienced in reflection when they have utilised this skill during training, albeit predominantly for academic assignments. However, facilitating such reflection in others requires very different skills (Gustafsson and Fagerberg, 2004). Learning through reflection in practice is fundamental with and demands various complex skills, such as foreseeing potential learning situations, articulating care components and making an assessment. Skill and experience are also required to uncover hidden practice through reflection otherwise expert nursing will remain silent.

Reflection before a situation requires skills in identifying the future pertinent, structured learning experiences that evolve from practice using intuition, clinical judgement and knowledge. Unless reflection occurs before a situation the process is restricted to single loop learning (Greenwood, 1998) as existing knowledge is not identified and therefore cannot be challenged. This highlights the need for leadership skills relating to workload prioritisation, seizing learning opportunities and creating an environment where students feel safe to question practice.

Reflection in practice necessitates proficient skills in articulating nursing and bringing out the rich components of care: this encompasses aesthetic knowledge and decision making (Johns, 1995). Without experience a mentor will have a small inventory of behaviours on which to act and respond, therefore limiting their synthesis from reflection (Fornasier, 2008). Inexperienced nurses adopt empirical, habitual practice that encourages confirmation, security and acceptance. It is only when care is deduced from empiricism to aesthetics that analysis occurs (Freshwater, 2004). Learning for inexperienced nurses is situationally based: their knowledge is not assimilated within the cognitive structures for storage and hence it cannot be recalled and applied to the various experiences that are generated from unpredictable healthcare events (Moon, 2007). Information that is lacking in meaning is discarded with only interpreted information being encoded and stored in the long-term memory, ready for recall (Welsh and Swann, 2002).

Experience involves the ability to 'be there' at the bedside, generating silent time and encoding information and the stimulation of thought (Ruth-Sahd and Tisdell, 2007). This silent time validates student practice and draws knowledge from a situation, thus creating new learning from reflection (Carr, 2005). The skills and confidence required for 'silent time' support the value of the intuition evolving from emotions and experiences gained over time and patient encounters. Emotions are registered before cognitive recognition (Ruth-Sahd and Tisdell, 2007), which is fundamental for reflection in action. A repertoire of emotions will stem from patient experiences and life experiences, with Schank

(Continued)

(Continued)

(1990) suggesting that nurses under the age of twenty-five lack the life skills necessary to deliver mature reflection. Experienced nurses will use multiple sources of knowledge, actively assimilating and connecting relevant information (termed discriminative reflectivity) (Mezirow, 1981). They are aware of the components embedded in care and possess the knowledge within these.

Reflecting on action involves undertaking critical analysis, exploring knowledge, and challenging assumptions and practice. This is often referred to as triple loop learning which during reflection converts into transformative learning where attitudes are re-organised, thereby promoting change (McAllister et al., 2005). Triple loop learning mirrors emancipatory reflection where constraints and habits are challenged, thus promoting autonomous beliefs (Taylor, 2006). Reflection on action provides opportunities to assess a student's knowledge and attitudes, with most teaching being conducted after patient care events (Field, 2004), and the mentor being accountable for the objective, valid and reliable assessment of student proficiency and competency. Assessment requires an in-depth knowledge of standards against which to measure, and therefore if the student is passed by a mentor who is an inexperienced practitioner then such judgements may ultimately have a detrimental effect on the nursing profession and patient care, with a potential adverse cycle being disseminated through professional hereditary.

Complex skills are required to unfold hidden practice and articulate care components, with reflection being a fundamental tool in linking theory to practice. The skills required to facilitate this learning effectively relate to Master's level knowledge and experience. Nurses are duty bound to protect the public and therefore the success of mentorship should be based upon the quality and not the quantity of mentors. Mentoring is a privilege and a position that should be earned: it is not a right or an imposition.

This case study certainly highlights some of the complexities of mentoring and the nature of the skills required by a mentor in order to facilitate reflection in others. The relatedness of expert practice and effective mentoring is clearly evident in Hall's reflection. The following table demonstrates the inter-connectedness of expertise in practice (Biggs, 2003), mentorship excellence (NMC, 2008; Health and Care Professions Council [HCPC], 2012;

Table 1.1 Mentor activity and Master's level practice characteristics

NMC domains	TCSW domains	HCPC standards (adapted)	Characteristics of a mentor	M-level practice characteristics
Establishing effective working relationships	Organise opportunities for the demonstration of assessed competence in practice	Provision of a safe, supportive environment	Model envisioner	Construct knowledge for themselves
Facilitation of learning	Enable learning and professional development in practice	Relevant knowledge, skills and experience	Energiser	Utilise appropriate disciplinary paradigms
Assessment and accountability	Manage the assessment of learners in practice	Provision of a range of learning and teaching methods that respects the rights and needs of service users	Investor	Recognise the insecure nature of knowledge
Evaluation of learning	Effective continuing performance as a practice educator	Learning, teaching and supervision that encourage safe and effective practice, independent learning and professional conduct	Supporter	Work more flexibly with ideas and arguments, enabling the suspension of judgements whilst evaluating contradictory alternatives
Creating an environment for learning	**(TCSW, 2012)**	Assessment of student performance must be objective and ensure fitness to practice	Career counsellor	**(Biggs, 2003)**
Context of practice		**(HCPC, 2012)**	Standard prodder	
Evidence-based practice			Teacher	
Leadership			Coach	
(NMC, 2008)			Feedback giver	
			Challenger	
			Eye opener	
			Door opener	
			Idea bouncer	
			Problem solver	
			(Darling, 1984)	

The College of Social Work [TCSW], 2012), and the seminal work of Darling (1984) which identifies the characteristics of an effective mentor.

When a mentor reflects on the above synthesis it becomes apparent that the integration of these fundamental mentoring activities occurs across professions and is underpinned by the characteristics of Master's level practice activity. It is this synthesis that demonstrates the mastery inherent within health and social care professional practice and mentorship. The mentoring activity of assessment and accountability is explicitly articulated across professional regulatory bodies' standards for practice education. This activity can be deconstructed, revealing the complexity of the activity in relation to Master's level practice activity (Biggs, 2003) and mentor characteristics (Darling, 1984). Biggs' descriptor relating to the ability to recognise the insecure nature of knowledge can be considered within the context of mentor characteristics, specifically those of standard prodder, feedback giver, challenger and door opener. A mentor is required to make judgements of professional competency in order to gate-keep the profession and ensure fitness to practice. They need to be highly skilled to facilitate assessment with sufficient flair and creativity in order to ensure that knowledge, skills and values are assessed in a balanced manner within professionally determined outcomes. Mentors can evaluate their mastery of assessment skills by referring to Benner's (1984) classic novice to expert model, in particular her description of a novice practitioner relying on external authorities as compared to an expert practitioner relying on internal authority. Given that mentors are experts within their professional field and in the advanced practice activity of mentorship they cannot merely rely on professionally determined criteria to assess competence. Rather they need to utilise their accumulated wisdom and internal authority to synthesise and evaluate divergent assessment information and thus ultimately make a judgement.

The final piece of this complex jigsaw is to consider the nature of Master's level academic descriptors and characteristics. The Quality Assurance Agency (2011) provides descriptors for all academic levels, including level seven Master's. The table below links these academic characteristics to key teaching and learning theoretical frameworks. It is evident that the Master's level characteristics relate to the higher order constructs within each of the frameworks. By virtue of their expertise in practice an effective mentor will be functioning at this higher level. Therefore mentors are in an ideal position to practise and study mentorship at Master's level.

Earlier we highlighted the integration of a range of mentor activities with Master's level characteristics (see Table 1.1) using assessment as an example of the practical application of this synthesis. Table 1.2 goes on to

Table 1.2 Overview of education models and academic levels

Academic level (QAA, 2011)	Bloom's taxonomy (1956) Cognitive domain	Affective domain	Psycho-motor domain	Anderson and Krathwohl (2001) Cognitive domain	Steinaker and Bell (1979) Experiential taxonomy	Benner (1984) Dreyfus model applied to nursing Competence
Master's characteristics (level 7 study)						
• Systematic understanding	Evaluation	Characteristics by value or value concept	Naturalisation	Creating	Dissemination	Expert
• Originality in application	Synthesis	Organising and conceptualising	Articulation	Evaluating	Internalisation	Proficient
• Deal with complex issues with creativity						
• Act autonomously						
• Demonstrate self-direction and originality						
• Exercise initiative and personal responsibility						
• Make decisions in complex and unpredictable situations						
Level 6 characteristics						
• Systematic understanding	Analysis	Valuing	Precision	Analysing	Identification	Competent
• Devise and sustain arguments	Application	Responding	Manipulation	Applying	Participation	Advanced beginner
• An appreciation of uncertainty and ambiguity	Comprehension	Receiving	Imitation	Understanding	Exposure	Novice
• Critically evaluate arguments	Knowledge			Remembering		
• Communicate information and ideas						
• Exercise initiative and personal responsibility						

demonstrate that Master's level characteristics are consistently reflected in the higher order constructs within key education theoretical models. When relating this to mentorship practice it is useful to once again consider the example of assessment, but this time specifically within the affective domain, and to focus on personal and professional values. Mentors should be able to demonstrate a conscious articulation of their own personal and professional values, role model these values effectively, and crucially should also be able to facilitate the identification of personal and professional values in their students. The skills required to do this are accurately reflected within both the QAA's level seven characteristics (2011) and the education models described. Mentors must possess a systematic understanding and intuitive grasp of the notion of values. If we take the example of a student nurse learning how to take a blood pressure early in the programme, that student will invariably focus on 'getting it right' and will concentrate on the cognitive and psycho motor domains. However, in this situation the mentor whilst needing to be able to assess these domains effectively is also required to explore the values underpinning the activity. They need to be able to deconstruct each of the domains and then situate these judgements within the context of values-based practice. This synthesis of assessment activity is highly complex and requires an ability to deal with uncertainty as well as demonstrate originality and creativity in the selection and application of assessment strategies.

Chapter summary

This chapter has been key to understanding the philosophy which drives the rest of the book. Mentorship is inherently an advanced practice activity and our argument is supported by the demonstration of the integration and synthesis of mentorship activities, Master's level practice characteristics, Master's characteristics and the higher construct orders that are evident in key education theories. The fact that mentors are practising mentorship at Master's level, coupled with key identified political, professional, economic and demographic drivers, indicates that mentorship preparation needs to be at Master's level. Mentors must recognise the mastery inherent within their mentorship practice, and should role model and share these skills along with celebrating the mentorship role as an advanced practice activity. The contribution of the various mentors in this book is an essential element to its success and highlights their own celebration of mentorship.

Reflective activity

After reading the chapter take a little time to consider the points below:

- Review in more detail the educational models presented in the chapter and consider their usefulness to the role of mentor.
- Reflect on an assessment you have undertaken with a student and consider the strategies you utilised in relation to Biggs' Master's practice characteristics.
- Write your own case study describing a mentorship scenario in your practice setting.

References

Anderson, L.W. and Krathwohl, D.R. (eds) (2001) *A Taxonomy for Learning, Teaching and Assessing: A Revision of Bloom's Taxonomy of Educational Objectives* (complete edition). New York: Longman.

Benner, P. (1984) *From Novice to Expert: Promoting Excellence and Power in Clinical Nursing Practice.* Menlo Park, CA: Addison-Wesley.

Biggs, J. (2003) *Teaching for Quality Learning at University* (2nd edn). Buckingham: SRHE and the Open University Press.

Bloom B.S. (1956) *Taxonomy of Educational Objectives, Handbook I: The Cognitive Domain.* New York: David McKay & Co Inc.

Carr, S. (2005) 'Knowing nursing – the challenge of articulating knowing in practice', *Nurse Education in Practice,* 5: 333–339.

Darling, L.A.W. (1984) 'What do nurses want in a mentor?', *Journal of Nursing Administration,* 14 (10): 42–44.

Field, D. (2004) 'Moving from novice to expert – the value of learning in clinical practice: a literature review', *Nurse Education Today,* 24: 560–565.

Fornasier, D. (2008) 'Teaching ethical leadership through the use of critical incident analysis', *Creative Nursing,* 14 (3): 116–122.

Freshwater, D. (2004) 'Analysing interpretation and re-interpreting analysis: exploring the logic of critical reflection', *Nursing Philosophy,* 5: 4–11.

Gainsbury, S. (2010) 'NMC acts on mentoring after *Nursing Times* mentors investigation'. Available at www.nursingtimes.net (last accessed 12 August 2012).

Greenwood, J. (1998) 'The role of reflection in single and double loop learning', *Journal of Advanced Nursing*, 27: 1048–1053.

Gustafsson, G. and Fagerberg, I. (2004) 'Reflection: the way to professional development', *Journal of Clinical Nursing*, 13: 271–280.

Health and Care Professions Council (2012) *Standards of Education and Training*. London: HCPC.

Johns, C. (1995) 'Framing learning through reflection within Carper's fundamental ways of knowing in nursing', *Journal of Advanced Nursing*, 22: 226–234.

McAllister, M., Tower, M. and Walker, R. (2005) 'Gentle interruptions: transformative approaches to clinical teaching', *Journal of Nursing Education*, 46: 304–312.

Mezirow, J. (1981) 'A critical theory of adult learning and education', *Adult Education*, 32 (1): 3–24.

Moon, J. (2007) *Reflection in Learning and Professional Development*. London: RoutledgeFalmer.

Neary, M. (2000) 'Supporting students' learning and professional development through the process of continuous assessment and mentorship', *Nurse Education Today*, 20: 463–474.

Nettleton, P. and Bray, L. (2008) 'Current mentorship scheme might be doing our students a disservice', *Nurse Education in Practice*, 8: 205–212.

Nursing and Midwifery Council (2008) *Standards to Support Learning and Assessment in Practice*. London: NMC.

Nursing and Midwifery Council (2010) *Standards for Pre-registration Nursing Education*. London: NMC.

Quality Assurance Agency (2011) *UK Quality Code for Higher Education*. Gloucester: QAA.

Ruth-Sahd, L. and Tisdell, E. (2007) 'The meaning and use of intuition in novice nurses: a phenomenological study', *Adult Education Quarterly*, 57 (2): 115–140.

Schank, M. (1990) 'Wanted: nurses with critical thinking skills', *Journal of Continuing Education in Nursing*, 21 (2): 86–89.

Shardlow, S. (2012) 'Learning and teaching in practice learning'. In J. Lishman (ed.) *Social Work Education and Training*. London: Jessica Kingsley.

Steinaker, N. and Bell, M. (1979) *The Experiential Taxonomy: A New Approach to Teaching and Learning*. New York: Academic Press.

Taylor, B. (2006) *Reflective Practice* (2nd edn). Milton Keynes: Open University Press.

The College of Social Work (2012) *Practice Educator Professional Standards for Social Work*. London: TCSW.

Welsh, I. and Swann, C. (2002) *Partners in Learning*. Oxford: Radcliffe Medical Press.

2 Establishing Effective Working Relationships

Case studies: Ian Stuart, Fiona Smith and Niina Alho

Across health and social care professional practice education, the emphasis on and the accepted notion of the value of an effective working relationship between mentors and pre-registration health and social care students are incontrovertible. Health and social care practice placements are complex and multifaceted environments as opposed to the relative comfort of the classroom. In practice students are exposed to patients/clients and their families/carers and friends, a core and wider team including numerous professionals and many others who input into patients'/clients' care and the practice arena. From a mentor's perspective they have a responsibility to socialise students into the reality of practice as well as the community of practice and contextualise, facilitate and support students' learning. The effectiveness of the relationship between mentor and student is vital to that student's learning experience and professional development. The development of an effective working relationship demands some recognition of its complexities on the part of the mentor and the employment of a range of skills in order to meet the challenges of that relationship. The benefits of effective working relationships between mentors and students are far reaching and will positively affect students, mentors, the practice area, the learning organisation, the health and social care professions, and crucially patient/client care.

This chapter will consider effective working relationships within health and social care practice education and will highlight the key influences on the development and maintenance of successful mentor–mentee relationships. Students consistently identify that the relationship with their mentor is the overriding factor in determining the extent to which they will both enjoy and learn from their practice placement. The attributes that make a good mentor will be examined in the context of effective working relationships, along with the concepts of role modelling and role conflict. The importance of providing a balance of informal and formal mentoring will be highlighted within the context of contemporary practice education and the potential challenges this presents to mentors and students.

Ian Stuart, the first case study author, is a social worker based within a mental health team. He explores the adoption of various aspects of a coaching model in order to enhance his mentorship skills. The second case study author, Fiona Smith, is a registered nurse in an operating department who describes the importance of establishing a good relationship early on in a placement. This is particularly important when practice placements are of a short duration. Smith identifies the specific characteristics mentors need to possess and highlights the role conflict that mentors have between the informal and formal aspects of mentoring and the tension within the relationship that these diverse roles may generate. The third case study author is Niina Alho, who is a registered nurse and mentor in a critical care environment. Alho reflects on a mentoring situation involving an experienced registered nurse who was, however, new to the critical care setting. She describes how the mentoring of this nurse was unsuccessful and identifies some of the influencing factors which had a negative impact.

The importance of the mentorship role in offering quality support to students is widely recognised and emphasised within health and social care practice education (Nursing and Midwifery Council [NMC], 2008; Health and Care Professions Council [HCPC], 2012; The College of Social Work [TCSW], 2012). Managing the complexities and challenges of establishing and maintaining effective working relationships requires mentors to employ higher level skills. This chapter will therefore examine those skills in relation to key aspects that are either identified within the case studies or evolved from them.

Chapter learning objectives

By the end of the chapter the reader should be able to:

- deconstruct the key features of an effective working relationship;
- critically evaluate the influences impacting on the development and maintenance of successful working relationships;
- critically reflect upon the concept of role modelling and the application of these skills in relation to this vital aspect of the mentoring role.

Defining effective working relationships within health and social care

When reviewing the multi-disciplinary literature across health and social care pertaining to the significance and value of effective working relationships between qualified experienced practitioners and students, there is much commonality to be discovered. An effective working relationship can be defined as a supportive, developmental and learning relationship between a mentor and mentee, one that is based on mutual respect and trust in which a novice student acquires and assimilates the appropriate knowledge, values, skills and professional behaviours that are required to enter their chosen profession. Grater-Nakamura et al. (2010) suggest that an effective working relationship within mentorship is a focused and complex developmental one that demands considerable commitment from both mentor and mentee. The importance of the learning environment within practice education is indisputable; however, research by Gray and Smith (2000) identified that students felt that the student–mentor relationship was just as crucial as the learning environment. In this longitudinal research students identified that a mentor's qualities, attitudes and skills were as important and influential in facilitating their learning and having a positive practice placement as the learning environment itself. Morton-Cooper and Palmer (2000) describe the mentoring relationship as one that fosters the empowerment of the student and is enabling within the practice area. It appears that at the heart of effective mentorship is the existence of an effective working relationship between the mentor and mentee. Therefore mentors need a comprehensive range of personal attributes and characteristics along with highly developed interpersonal skills in order to establish and maintain effective working relationships. In this first case study Ian Stuart, a social worker, describes how he used a coaching model to develop his mentoring skills. The coaching model emphasises some of the key skills needed by the mentor in order to facilitate an effective and productive relationship between learner and mentor. The use of self and effective questioning skills is emphasised within the model. Stuart argues that this approach is particularly useful for postgraduate students as it emphasises learner autonomy and responsibilities.

Chapter link

What are the characteristics of an effective learning environment? (See Chapter 6 for more information.)

CASE STUDY

Using the coaching model in developing professional knowledge and competence in postgraduate learning – Ian Stuart

Facilitating learning in the practice setting for postgraduate students can present the practice teacher/mentor with specific challenges. It can also be extremely rewarding for the educator and the team involved. I am a social worker working in a community mental health team and I have supported a range of postgraduate learners within this environment, ranging from those on post-qualifying awards such as Approved Mental Health Practitioner (AMHP) to others working towards an MA in Applied Mental Health Practice. In my experience these students have often come to the practice setting with a wide range of life and learning experiences, and, to paraphrase an old quote, 'Sometimes it's not learning new behaviours that is the problem, it's getting rid of old ones'. I have found it important to be aware of each student's past learning and how this has been applied in practice and also the current learning needs of that student. Eraut (1994) makes the point that it can be difficult to transfer knowledge from one context to another without considerable further learning taking place. My dilemma in these situations has been how to ensure that this significant previous learning and experience can be used to facilitate learning within my specific environment. I have found the coaching model devised by Whitmore (2009) to be an extremely useful paradigm in which to develop knowledge and learning as well as a safe method by which to manage the subjective experiences of students.

What is coaching?

Coaching is about learning throughout life in a natural and positive way. As human beings we want to learn, we love to explore, we have an innate desire to grow and develop, and we are naturally curious. Coaching engages that curiosity and there are several models of coaching all of which share the same basic principles and aims (Thorpe and Clifford, 2003; Claridge and Lewis, 2005). Over the last decade increasing attention has been paid to the possibility of coaching models being used as a basis for the development of skills and increasing performance based on self-awareness and responsibility (Drake, 2008). Coaching has its foundations in a multi-dimensional model of human development and communication that has drawn from the best of humanistic, positive and integral psychology (Williams, 2008). It also draws heavily on adult learning theory, systems theory and organisational development, and has philosophical roots in constructivism and existentialism (Tennant, 2006).

Coaching is not a therapeutic approach, but it does use some theoretical concepts and evidence-based practices that have been developed in various recognised schools of therapeutic intervention, such as cognitive behavioural therapy and solution-focused therapy. The nature of the relationship between mentor and mentee is a crucial element within the coaching relationship. A conversation between two people is as old as the dawn of time and a natural human activity (De Shazer, 1994). It is our opportunity to, among other things, pass on information, test out theories, obtain feedback and reflect, which in turn will influence our social functioning and learning.

The coaching conversation highlights these issues and helps develop a 'cognitive space' in which the adult learner is able to consider their goals in a contextual format (Thorpe and Clifford, 2003).

Coaching is about uncovering what people want (their goals) and their core values, and then supporting them to be aware of their own resourcefulness and skills in order to make the changes they desire. It helps develop focus and when we focus on something we will usually attain it. The coach or mentor will facilitate the learner to generate their own solutions and ultimately the responsibility is on the learner to generate results. The past

(Continued)

(Continued)

need not dictate the future. A coach needs to listen to and acknowledge an individual's story and past experiences, but having done so they will support that person in creating new stories and unlock their true potential by taking action (Kim-Berg and Szabo, 2005).

A coach will facilitate this process with effective listening skills, hearing what is being said and reflecting it back; with effective questioning and asking open questions, making people think; with building trust and a rapport; with promoting awareness, responsibility and self-belief; and with encouraging the ability to summarise and develop action plans. Using the G.R.O.W. model (Whitmore, 2009), the coaching process helps learners to identify and set clear goals, i.e. 'What do you want specifically?' (Goal). It explores the current situation, i.e. 'What is happening? What action have you taken so far?' (Reality). It will also explore other potential strategies and alterative courses of action, i.e. 'What are the options available to you? What else?' (Options). Finally, it will look at what is to be done, when and by whom i.e. 'What will you do? Will this action meet your goal? What obstacles might you face? Can these be dealt with? What degree of certainty do you have that you will carry out the actions agreed (Willingness/ way forward)?' This is followed by an agreed plan, a time-scale, and other outcome measures (adapted from Whitmore, 2009).

Coaching is non-analytical; the content of the coaching conversation does not need to be reinterpreted in terms of some other psychological model. It is not mutually exclusive; the coaching model can be used as an overall framework and does allow for other models to co-exist, and it can complement others – particularly adult learning (Tennant, 2006). Coaching also minimises attachment or dependency issues (Foster-Turner ,2006) as it helps develop self-reliance by increasing personal awareness and responsibility.

The Coach

Through the use of his/her experience, expertise and encouragement a coach can help a learner achieve specific goals. The coach's aim is to build trust and rapport as he/she acts as a collaborative partner, in order to develop the skills and knowledge that are needed to improve the learner's professional career. The coach uses goal setting, action planning, questioning skills (ask, don't tell), active listening and behavioural change techniques.

The development of a rapport between coach and learner is a high priority in coaching and essential to creating a supportive learning environment. O'Conner and Lages (2004) and Henwood and Lister (2007) argue that the importance of this rapport should not be underestimated and efforts to reach 'peak rapport' will have a major impact on the learner attaining their goals and transforming their thinking and behaviour. The aim is to assist people in developing their skills, knowledge and understanding through identifying their goals and how to achieve them; this involves a process of thinking and the development of a cognitive space which will allow students to consider how they will behave or what actions they may take in certain situations.

In my experience coaching has proved to be a useful model when facilitating learning in the practice environment. It reminds me that coaching or mentoring is about engaging in a conversation with students where I have to listen actively, take note of any assumptions and then check these assumptions out. I then need to speak honestly and openly after I have listened closely. I need to remember to use effective questions in order to raise awareness and responsibility within learners. I must also remember to adopt an 'ask, don't tell' approach as this encourages learning, summarising what I think is being said and always giving feedback. This positive process can help to prevent unnecessary conflict between mentors and students and is an exciting way to facilitate learning.

Characteristics of an effective mentor

In research undertaken by Myall et al. (2008) students identified the qualities they looked for in a mentor. These qualities included being supportive, knowledgeable, enthusiastic, helpful, experienced and committed to their role as a mentor. The students also cited the quality of the relationship between themselves and their mentor as important and articulated that a good relationship was based on mutual understanding and respect. A multitude of key characteristics are posited across health and social care practice education as being essential for both effective mentoring and effective relationships and these can be summarised as follows.

Effective mentors should possess attributes relating to: patience, respect, a sense of humour, knowledge, enthusiasm (Fawcett, 2002); effective interpersonal skills, an approachable manner, good teaching and supervision skills (Andrews and Wallis, 1999); honesty, sincerity, empathy, caring, political awareness, analytical and critical thinking skills, professional expertise, skills in giving positive and constructive feedback (Grater-Nakamura et al., 2010); and appropriate role modelling skills (Anderson, 2011). Gopee (2011: 33) also offers a useful collective of characteristics identified by students that a mentor is required to possess:

- is patient;
- open-minded;
- approachable;
- has a good knowledge base;
- knowledge and competence are up to date;
- has good communication skills including listening skills;
- provides encouragement;
- is self-motivated;
- shows concern, compassion and empathy;
- provides psychological support;
- acts as a counsellor;
- is tactful;
- diplomatic, fun and fair;
- willing to be a mentor;
- versatile, adaptable and flexible;
- allows time and commits self to it;
- is confident;
- enthusiastic;
- acts as an advisor;
- is honest and trustworthy;
- trusting;
- acts as a role model;
- is non-judgemental;
- is a resource facilitator;
- is able to build working relationships

Key work undertaken by Darling in 1984 is frequently cited in the current literature pertaining to mentorship. Following a two-year study exploring the characteristics nurses valued in their mentors and needed to be evident in order to meet their expectations of the mentor–mentee relationship, Darling identified three absolute requirements for effective mentoring. These characteristics were mutual respect, mutual attraction, and the commitment of time and energy. Darling articulated the mentor role within 14 parameters, these being role model, envisioner, energiser, investor, supporter, standard-prodder, teacher-coach, feedback-giver, eye-opener, door-opener, idea bouncer, problem solver, career counsellor and challenger.

Several authors offer descriptions of how Darling's characteristics for mentorship are demonstrated within the mentorship role and effective working relationships with students (Morton-Cooper and Palmer, 2000; West et al., 2007; Gopee, 2011). In the case study in Chapter 5 Bailey-McHale discusses the use of these characteristics to enable mentors to evaluate the effectiveness of their mentorship. Mentors and student mentors may find the following eclectic descriptions of Darling's characteristics for mentorship useful, and when seen as a model or approach to mentorship they can be considered in the context of the more recent NMC's (2008) eight domains in the standards for mentoring.

Table 2.1 Characteristics of effective mentors

Role Model	The importance of being a positive role model cannot be overemphasised. The mentor should be someone who the student can look up to, admire and respect. By role modelling appropriately, the mentor should provide 'an observable image demonstrating skills and qualities for the student to emulate' (Morton-Cooper and Palmer, 2000: 43). As a positive role model the mentor consistently practises an excellent standard of nursing, demonstrating current knowledge and skills including decision-making skills in their practice arena. Their practice is patient/client centred, taking opportunities to discuss plans and options for care with the patient/client/families within an ethical framework. The mentor is clearly committed to and enthusiastic about being a mentor.
Envisioner	The mentor is able to enable the student to make sense of practice in a creative manner, including the ability to see opportunities for care/intervention options beyond the immediate. Care/intervention considerations are cognisant of patient/client empowerment. The mentor is innovative and looks for ways to improve care.
Energizer	The mentor is enthusiastic about interactions with patients/clients, demonstrating to the student opportunities to communicate with patients/clients and reassess their needs. The mentor should encourage the student to move beyond a task-focused approach to care and motivate the student to be inspired and enthusiastic about the scope of professional practice.
Investor	The mentor commits to spending time with the student, recognising and valuing the student's abilities and working with them to develop their practice. The mentor trusts the student and delegates to them appropriately, spending time feeding back to the student and encouraging them to reflect on their own practice and that of the mentor.

(Continued)

Table 2.1   (Continued)

Supporter	The mentor is friendly, warm and caring towards the student and supportive of them as they are exposed to practice situations. The mentor provides the student with both personal and professional support in order for that student to learn and develop as a professional.
Challenger	The mentor encourages the student to explore their own beliefs, values and opinions which may influence their professional practice. The mentor appropriately questions the student regarding their beliefs, values and opinions, thereby facilitating them to examine their decisions and develop critical thinking skills.
Standard Prodder	The mentor has current knowledge and clarity relating to the standard of competence and level of achievement that is required of students in practice at all stages of the professional education programme each student is undertaking. The mentor motivates the student to achieve the required standard and assesses whether or not they have attained the required level of achievement. The mentor is confident of their own competence and readily questions their own practice and that of the student.
Teacher and Coach	The mentor shares their knowledge and experience with the student, teaching the craft of practice underpinned by evidence. The mentor identifies the student's learning needs along with the student and provides opportunities for learning through experience.
Feedback Giver	The mentor is able to give positive, constructive and timely feedback, enabling the student to build on achievements, explore situations where practice could have been improved and identify learning needs. The mentor provides regular formative feedback, allowing the student time and opportunities to achieve competence. The mentor observes interactions between the student and patients/clients, and reflects on and critiques these interactions with the student.
Eye Opener	The mentor exposes the student to and inspires interest in the macro factors that influence health and social care. Examples are research, governmental policy, national guidance, corporate governance and local organisational systems of care, policy and guidelines.
Door Opener	The mentor encourages and guides the student to identify wider resources for learning, including other health and social care professionals. The mentor actively includes the student in intra- and multi-professional team discussions and facilitates the student's networking.
Idea Bouncer	The mentor demonstrates a willingness and openness to discuss and debate complexities of care and wider issues, encouraging the student to formulate and contribute new ideas and approaches. The mentor will allow time for the student to reflect on their extended thinking.

Problem solver	The mentor is patient with the student who is attempting to problem solve and facilitates their problem-solving abilities by promoting the development of student skills relating to critical thinking, critical analysis and decision making.
Educational Counsellor	The mentor is a trusted practitioner who is able to give a considered opinion and guidance to the student regarding career planning. The mentor understands and supports the student's aspirations to succeed in their chosen health and social care profession.

Role modelling

The public has a right to expect high standards of health and social care provision. In order to meet societies', professional regulatory bodies' and students' expectations mentors need to be excellent role models, practising and representing their profession to a very high standard. Paice et al. (2002), when considering good medical role models for junior doctors, asserted that a good role model is someone we can identify with, who has the qualities we would like to have and is in a position we would like to be in. Common to definitions of a role model is the notion that a role model facilitates the transfer of evidence-based practice, appropriate professional values and behaviours, and experiential insights to students. Based on Bandura's (1977) social learning theory relating to role modelling it is assumed that students will emulate the practice of their mentors. Of course it is vital that mentors role model appropriately; however, Grealish and Ranse (2009) point out that students don't merely emulate all of their mentors' practice and are discerning enough not to replicate undesirable values or practice. Effective mentors will role model excellent practice and professional behaviour to their students whilst encouraging them to develop their own ways of practising. When immersed in the chaos and complexity of professional practice students have many opportunities to observe their mentors engaging and interacting with patients/clients whilst delivering care or undertaking interventions. An effective mentor will explain the rationale for the care given and role model the appropriate behaviour knowing that there is more than one right way to deliver care. When considering social-work education Ruch (2012) argued the need for professional practitioners to possess the ability to demonstrate professional vulnerability. This vulnerability provides students with examples of the need to think critically and reflectively about practice in order to achieve professional competence. By facilitating students to apply theory to practice and learn by doing, mentors will encourage them to develop their own appropriate style of practice.

Chapter link

How does Bandura's social learning theory relate to other key learning approaches? (See Chapter 3 for more information.)

It is also important for mentors and student mentors to extend their thinking by considering themselves as role models in the context of the wider organisation and potential future mentors. Mentors need to contribute to the values and mission of their organisation, challenging where necessary in order to foster a positive learning organisation. By role modelling the organisation's agreed vision a mentor can demonstrate how a shared understanding of collaborative goals can improve patient/client care. Facilitating student awareness of the shared mission of the organisation can help students feel part of the broader health and social care arena and develop their understanding relating to their accountability to their employer. Relating to the development of future mentors, Melincavage (2011) asserts that student nurses learn more than patient care and clinical skills, they also learn about the ways qualified staff relate to students. If students are consistently exposed to poor mentoring they may be in danger of believing that elements of a mentor's treatment of students are normal behaviour. This may then adversely affect their relationships with students when they become the mentors of tomorrow. Student nurses have identified that towards the end of their programme they not only think about their role as a registered nurse but also about their future role as a mentor and how they would act as a role model (Gray and Smith, 2000). These students based their thoughts regarding their future roles on their mentoring experiences throughout their practice education, citing how mentors who were positive role models and enthusiastic about nursing as a profession gave them hope for the future. Medical students also rank a positive attitude towards junior colleagues and students as one of the most important qualities of a positive role model (Paice et al., 2002). Students clearly identify that mentors have an influential role in helping to form their perceptions about how they will function as mentors, thereby adding to the evidence of the importance of role modelling. In the following case study, through her experience of mentoring a student on a short placement, Fiona Smith identifies several pertinent issues, including the importance of establishing effective relationships with students and role conflict.

Establishing effective relationships – Fiona Smith

In the operating department, where placements can last for as little as two weeks and as long as eight weeks, the early establishment of an effective mentor–mentee relationship is vital. Over the past ten to fifteen years the operating department has not always been included within the pre-registration nursing programme. To ensure that the student nurse is exposed to the complexities of the operating department it is vital that they are allocated a placement. This will encourage an interest within the student in the operating department and could have a positive effect on their potential recruitment. Not all our students are nurses; they do however make up the predominant numbers, along with medical students and paramedic students. This case study was based upon the establishment of a relationship with a student nurse in order to facilitate learning within a positive practice placement.

I have found that the best placements are achieved when the learning takes place in an informal atmosphere and combines theory as well as 'hands-on' practice. This is a view reinforced by Ali and Panther (2008) and Sharp et al. (2006) who suggest a mentor should encompass the following roles: advisor, coach, counsellor, guide, role model, sponsor, teacher and resource facilitator. Student assessment is also recognised as a vital aspect of the mentor's role. It is vital that a mentor has the requisite skills and knowledge to effectively undertake assessment. This may be difficult for someone to achieve alongside all of the other identified roles of a mentor. Gopee (2011) reinforces these concerns by suggesting mentors may not be competent to assess students, as such an assessment requires the ability to recognise, confront and analyse both ethical and clinical situations, a role that may directly conflict with the other aspects of mentorship.

It is important to consider the characteristics required of mentors in order to successfully manage the diversity of roles. These characteristics include friendliness, a sense of humour, patience, approachability and good interpersonal skills, professional development combined with mutual respect, empathy, environmental understanding and co-operation, all of which must be combined with the ability to support students. On reflection, when considering my roles and responsibilities as a mentor, this list of roles and required characteristics appears somewhat overwhelming. This reflection encouraged me to consider in more detail the importance of

(Continued)

(Continued)

building an effective relationship quickly in order to balance the assessment aspects of the mentorship role with its more traditional aspects.

I was aware when preparing for my student that the development of the initial relationship is crucial, particularly as the operating department can be an alien environment to many students. Unfortunately, due to departmental re-structuring, I was unable to meet with my student prior to her arrival. However I did ensure that I was on duty on her first day. Ali and Panther (2008) remind us that the pressure of both time and work commitments can prevent the development of a supportive relationship. Steinaker and Bell (1979) also argue that the initial development of a strong relationship will encourage intellectual commitment.

Our busy operating department can seem chaotic to new students and this can also have an effect on mentors and their ability to form relationships and structure learning. I was keen to ensure that our initial meeting established a sense of belonging and safety. This meant that I had to consider the constraints of the environment whilst also ensuring that the student could indeed learn. Eps et al. (2006) argue from student feedback that the mentors who were perceived to facilitate professional development were the ones who provided opportunities for practice. In other words, they provided the appropriate level of support for students to develop within the clinical area. Without this support there is no feeling of belonging and some students will develop diminished motivation, which will inevitably lead to an unsatisfactory placement for both mentor and mentee. I tried to ensure that I managed my workload demands without too much impact on the student's learning by including them in what I was doing, discussing with them what I was thinking and asking them for their opinion.

Empathy is a quality usually reserved for patients. I would argue, however, that it should also be shared with colleagues, whether this is in the form of acceptance or inclusion within the team. It was identified as one of the four most crucial aspects identified by students in a study by Edwards et al. (2004). Sharing a common understanding is an important aspect of the whole placement experience. By investing time into ensuring both my student and I had a shared understanding of what was expected, particularly in terms of learning outcomes, the complexities of the assessment role were managed effectively. This involved forward planning and an understanding of my student's requirements. To achieve this I arranged structured, regular meetings in which we would discuss, without preconceptions, the development of the placement and their ongoing requirements. Acknowledging shared interests and common ground between the mentor and mentee can also be effective at the start of a relationship. Darling (1985) and Andrews and

Wallis (1999) go as far as suggesting that when mentors and protégés have the same world view this can provide significant opportunities, facilitate learning, and integrate both theory and practice.

Humour is an under-reported area within practice learning and yet it is identified in many of the lists regarding the characteristics of a good mentor. It can supply the building blocks on which a good relationship is based. There are, however, some dangers inherent with the use of humour within practice learning and mentors need to be conscious of the nature and content of the humour. Equally it can be used positively to alleviate stress and tension and this can be vital in a short-term placement. It is important that a mentor never uses humour in a negative manner. I was able to use humour with my student appropriately and I was also pleased that the student could take part in the general banter within the operating department.

Mentors currently need to manage these diverse roles; however, some have suggested that the mentor role and the assessor role should be separated. Arguably mentor preparation programmes still leave many people unclear about their responsibilities due to the dichotomy of the roles between supporting and assessing, and this is further compounded by the limited time-frame available to mentors within many placements. Combining the role of supportive mentor and assessor is a difficult task and separating the two roles would simplify the practice experience. However, who could be in a better position to unpick the skills required to nurse effectively than a nurse working alongside a student?

Role conflict

There has been much debate concerning the potential confusion that may occur regarding the terminology used to describe those professionals who guide and support students and assess their competence within health and social care professional practice education. For example, the term 'practice assessor' is used in social work and the term 'mentor' in nursing and midwifery. This confusion, whilst having potential implications for inter-professional mentorship, does not detract from the clarity we have moved towards regarding two key features of practice education. Firstly, mentorship is accepted as an effective model for supporting, guiding and supervising students across health and social care professions, with its attendant significant responsibility in determining fitness to practice. Secondly, whatever the title, the complexity and diverse nature of the role is common across health and social care professions and firmly embedded. Within nursing and midwifery an amalgamated mentorship role has been clearly articulated for over a decade and is reflected in the still current and widely quoted definition produced by the English National Board for Nursing, Midwifery and Health Visiting in 2001. The ENB's definition is 'The term mentor is used to denote the role of the nurse, midwife or health visitor who facilitates learning and supervises and assesses students in the practice setting' (ENB, 2001: 6). The benefits of effective mentorship for both mentors and mentees are well established and are summarised in Table 2.2.

Evidently for mentors being able to role model and share their expertise with students, and observe them moving towards achieving the competence required for professional practice, is highly beneficial. Being instrumental in guiding, supporting and assessing students must be rewarding; however,

Table 2.2 The benefits of mentoring for the mentor and student

Benefits for mentors	Benefits for students
• an increased sense of job satisfaction; • a sense of pride through observing students develop their knowledge skills and professional attitudes (Myall et al., 2008); • development of communication and interpersonal skills; • enhancement of leadership skills; • development of new insights into own practice; • increased contribution to innovation and new ideas; • increased contribution to professional networking and the development of colleagues; • increased contribution to the meeting of quality assurance goals (Grater-Nakamura et al., 2010); • increased learning skills; • a greater awareness and access to educational programmes; • potential career enhancement; • being energised by meaningful discussions and reflections and reciprocal learning (Sword et al., 2002); • increased connection with the theoretical basis of professional practice programmes (Huybrecht et al., 2011).	• being welcomed to the practice placement and team and treated with respect as a valued learner (Kinnel and Hughes, 2010); • being supported throughout the placement and helped to feel connected to the practice area and team; • being given appropriate and timely opportunities to maximise learning; • development of increased confidence in their professional role and autonomy; • development of increased self-esteem (Grater-Nakamura et al., 2010); • development of decision-making skills; • encouragement to explore interpersonal dilemmas; • time and guidance to reflect on practice, including organisational, legal and ethical factors.

mentors have various challenges in relation to managing role conflict. As identified by Smith in her case study, mentors have to deal with role conflict in relation to having multiple roles outside of their mentorship role and multiple roles within the mentorship role. Mentors are required to manage an ever-changing and dynamic multiplicity of roles along with their mentorship role and these are likely to present them with competing priorities. There are several key challenges to the mentorship role identified and reiterated across the health and social care professional education literature. These include time constraints as the result of busy clinical workloads, coupled with inadequate staffing levels, inconsistent ongoing support for the mentorship role and too many students being placed in the practice area, along with limited resources for education. Key work undertaken by Phillips et al. (2000) explored common role conflicts for mentors, an adaptation of which is presented below in Table 2.3.

More recent research undertaken by Carlisle et al. (2009) identified from a mentor survey, nurse mentors' views regarding key aspects of a mentor's role and barriers to their ability to effectively undertake this role. These important aspects and barriers are illustrated below in Table 2.4, with the most frequently cited features occurring at the top of each list.

Table 2.3 Role conflict for mentors

The mentor as a registered professional delivering care	Role conflict may arise from: • the competing priorities between delivering care, including the organisation and delegation of care, and supporting, teaching, observing and assessing the student; • when the dynamic nature of the practice arena determines that the mentor has to give care in a different place from where the student is engaged in practice.
The mentor as a manager	• the competing priorities of the organisation who may require the mentor to manage the practice area, a team or a particular situation as well as mentor the student; • the interruption of mentoring the student in order to undertake management activities; • time away from the student's practice setting in order to undertake management or organisational functions.
The mentor as a student	• the mentor may be undertaking an educational programme themselves including a mentorship preparation programme. The mentor may experience competing priorities between their own learning needs and those of their student. This may cause particular difficulty when the underlying philosophy of the mentor's assessment is different from that of the assessment of the student that the mentor is supporting.

Table 2.4 Important aspects of and potential barriers to the mentor's role

Important aspects of the mentor role:	Potential barriers to the mentor role:
• supervision of students undertaking skills; • welcoming students to the practice environment and helping them to feel valued; • planning a programme of learning for each student; • collaboratively working with students; • creating opportunities for students to learn from others; • assessing students' practice; • providing feedback to students; • providing sufficient opportunities for students to reflect on their experiences; • familiarising oneself with the students' programme including assessments; • helping to reduce students' stress; • introducing students to the wider team.	• conflict of interest due to the demands of clinical care; • conflict of interest due to the demands of clinical management; • lack of recognition by managers of the demands of the role; • working within the constraints of the documentation; • own lack of understanding of the students' curriculum; • lack of support from clinical colleagues.

The main resource issue acting as a barrier to effective mentoring appears to be a scarcity of time. Managers, colleagues and mentors themselves may underestimate the energy, responsibility and commitment required to undertake the role, including the availability of protected time with the student. Other members of the health and social care team may perceive that time spent with a student takes the mentor away from other activities, thereby increasing the workload of other team members. It is not always accepted that workloads should be distributed in such a way as to recognise those who are mentoring and those who are not. Rather than support their mentor colleagues other team members may resent what they see as unequal workloads, leaving the mentor feeling unsupported or worse isolated and adding to the role conflict the mentor experiences. Carlson et al. (2009) assert that the managers of practice areas find it difficult to increase the workload of some staff in order to allow mentors sufficient time to mentor effectively. Therefore some mentors have to manage and balance mentoring alongside their other roles with no real reduction of their workload. Professional regulatory bodies do recognise and stipulate the necessity of protected time for mentors and mentees (NMC, 2008; HCPC, 2012), however consistently applying these standards in the professional practice arena continues to be problematic.

Mentors can employ a number of strategies to improve their support in the practice area, utilising highly developed interpersonal, negotiation, leadership and role modelling skills. They will also have been educated as to the

importance of the learning environment for students and of involving others, including their managers, in regularly reviewing the learning environment to generate collegial support. This team inclusiveness in improving the
practice learning environment not only for students but for the whole practice team and patients/clients will inspire enthusiasm for students and increase
understanding of the mentoring role. Allocating two mentors to each student
or adopting a team mentorship approach can also negate some of the time
constraint issues by maximising learning opportunities and allowing for
greater flexibility in the organisation of care and workloads. A further potential strategy is one recently witnessed by the author of this chapter. A stage
two nurse mentor contacted me as the link lecturer for her practice area to
seek support whilst she facilitated an educational session with team colleagues who were registered practitioners and as such stage one mentors.
This nurse mentor noticed that colleagues seemed to be reluctant to spend
time with students. It appeared that these colleagues were unconfident as to
what they could offer these students. The mentor presented information
about the students' programme, reassured colleagues that appropriate feedback mechanisms would be in place and emphasised the value of their experience to the students' learning. Following the session and regular follow-up
meetings the mentor's colleagues now regularly facilitate students learning as
appropriate, with some wanting to extend their mentorship skills and responsibility by undertaking stage-two mentorship preparation. Primarily robust
systems for feedback are vital for the mentor and student both formatively
and summatively; however, this dialogue between mentors and other colleagues also serves to add value to the learning environment.

Chapter link

Can you explain the difference between formative and summative
assessments? (See Chapter 4 for more information.)

In contemporary health and social care practice education, mentors have
the dual role of traditional mentorship coupled with responsibility for
assessment. Smith, in her case study, describes the experience of this tension
between the traditional mentor role and that of assessor. Mentorship in the

context of its traditional meaning denotes a longer-term relationship, in which an experienced and wise person guides, supports, advises and befriends a more junior protégée or colleague in order to pass on their knowledge and experience. Smith poses the question of whether the two distinct aspects should be separated. Wilkes (2006) suggests that while the development of friendship between the mentor and student enhances the practice placement experience, the student's achievements may not be an accurate reflection of competency due to an element of subjectivity. Oft-cited research undertaken by Duffy (2004) raised concerns regarding the 'failure to fail', identifying some nurse mentors' reluctance to assess students as not being competent in practice environments. Participants revealed the emotional impact of failing students, describing the experience as traumatic and horrendous. Due to the complexity of the dual aspects of the role, mentors may experience the dilemma of the need to fail an unsafe student versus the difficulty in failing a 'friend' and potentially ending that student's professional ambitions. There is some debate as to whether the roles should be separated in order to minimise the stress that a mentor experiences when having to fail a student. Bray and Nettleton (2007) suggest that separating the roles of mentor and assessor should be given serious consideration in order to avoid role conflict. It can be argued that the tension between the mentor's role in supporting a student and assessing that individual can potentially undermine the mentor–student relationship. Diluting the supportive aspects of the mentorship role with an emphasis on assessment can lead to pseudomentoring. While there have been some initiatives that have explored the reconfiguring of the mentorship/assessing role it appears that the current prominent approach to mentoring with its multiple roles will continue into the foreseeable future. Huybrecht et al. (2011) suggest that mentors recognise all aspects of their role and see assessment as a crucial part of their overall role, and as long as a clear mentoring process is in place mentors are not confused by the remit of their role. Cavanagh (2002) asserts that it is the very complexity of the multiple roles within mentorship that makes it worthwhile. One of the inherent skills within professional practice is an ability to build effective therapeutic relationships with patients/clients, including making objective ongoing assessments of people's health and social care needs. Therefore it is likely that with appropriate support mentors can apply their transferrable skills to the current model of mentoring. Again it appears that time is a vital component for mentors to be able to balance the multiple roles within their mentorship role. Protected time for feedback, reflection and ongoing assessment is crucial for the mentor–student relationship and the latter's professional development. The importance of support for mentors from colleagues, managers and lecturing staff within the higher education institution (HEI) is already well documented (Watson, 2000; Myall et al., 2008; Huybrecht et al., 2011). Some suggested strategies are:

- access to mentorship preparation programmes and regular mentor updates;
- regular contact between the mentor and link lecturer, with the link lecturer visiting the practice area;
- a collaborative approach to managing a failing student, with the link lecturer supporting the mentor, student and wider team;
- collaboration between mentors, the link lecturer and practice placement manager regarding educational audits;
- the link lecturer ensuring the provision of information relating to professional regulatory bodies' standards and guidance for mentors: for example, in nursing and midwifery the requirement for a triennial review;
- access to Practice Education Facilitators (PEFs) who can support the mentor with a variety of student issues (Carlisle et al., 2009);
- organisational structures that recognise and value the mentor's role (Fisher and Webb, 2008).

It is evident that mentors require preparation and ongoing support in order to manage the conflicting roles and responsibilities demanded by the contemporary mentorship role. The organisation, managers, colleagues and lecturing staff from the HEI all need to contribute to facilitating the diverse nature of a mentor's role. The key factor in successful mentorship is the establishment of an effective working relationship.

Establishing and maintaining effective relationships

Fundamental to the quality of the learning experience for students and the mentoring process is the effectiveness of the mentor–student relationship. As Smith highlights in her case study, mentors may have students for relatively short periods of time and therefore need to establish a relationship early on in the placement. Barry (2009) identifies how daunting new practice placements can be and that the student's basic needs should be considered and met before higher level needs such as learning can be considered. Sharp et al. (2006) in their mentoring resource consider the start of the mentor–student relationship in the context of Maslow's (1987) 'Hierarchy of needs', and the following questions are an adaption of their ideas for mentors:

- Are your student's basic needs being met, including their psychological and physical comfort? For example, access to information as to when their breaks will be and where to get something to eat and drink – reflecting Maslow's physiological needs.
- Have you identified and addressed any fears or concerns your student may have? For example, any worries and unrealistic preconceived views regarding the nature of the practice area – reflecting Maslow's safety needs.
- Have you introduced the student to the team in order to foster their sense of value and belonging? For example, an introduction to the team and patients/clients will help them feel welcomed – reflecting Maslow's love and belongingness needs.
- Have you explored the student's personal motivation, prior learning and experience, and discussed any personal issues that may impact on their learning? – reflecting Maslow's self-esteem needs.
- Have you identified what interests and motivates the student professionally? – reflecting Maslow's self-actualisation needs.

Students report that feeling welcomed by their mentor and the team is vital for their practice placement learning experience. The initial meeting between student and mentor offers the mentor an ideal opportunity to foster trust. A meaningful induction to the practice area, including an introduction to multidisciplinary team members, will help the student to feel comfortable in the team and engage in practice activity. The initial meeting or meetings will serve several purposes which can positively affect the development of an effective working relationship. These purposes include:

- helping the mentor and student to get to know each other, identifying the mentor's and student's previous experience and the student's learning needs. Together the mentor and student can plan appropriate strategies and identify opportunities to facilitate the student's learning;
- mentors setting the boundaries of the relationship by discussing with the student both parties' expectations of the relationship. Whilst helping the student to understand that the mentor has many commitments, the mentor can reassure the student that they or other team members will be available and accessible to them. The mentor should then identify the supportive and assessment aspects of their role and

in doing so will both help the student to develop their awareness of personal and professional boundaries and help themself to manage role conflict;

- helping mentors to support students in their transition from one learning environment to another. For example, a social work student may be coming from a placement with a probation team working with adults in the community to gain experience with a hospital-based social work team focusing on discharge planning. Different learning environments are influenced by different organisational cultures, management styles and systems for the delivery of care.

In terms of maintaining an effective relationship there are recognised phases that the mentor–student relationship goes through. Firstly, there is the initiation phase in which the mentor and student are working together and closely observing each other. The mentor needs to offer the appropriate level of support, guidance and supervision in order for the student to practise and learn safely. The working phase comes next in which the student becomes more active as they become more confident in themselves, safe in their trusting relationship with their mentor. In this second phase the student takes on more responsibility for their learning and becomes more independent in practice. The final phase is the termination phase during which the relationship ends either positively or negatively (Morton-Cooper and Palmer, 2000). Hopefully the termination of the relationship will be positive, with the student successfully moving on in their professional education programme having gained confidence in their achievements and being able to apply and build on their learning in their next placement. A successful end to the relationship should leave the mentor with a greater sense of job satisfaction and sufficient enthusiasm for the next student. In many practice placements these phases will need to occur in a short period of time and will require the mentor to possess a range of skills to ensure the maintenance of an effective relationship throughout these phases. Grater-Nakamura et al. (2010) identify several key features of the effective working relationship which demand a high level of skill in order for the mentor to facilitate multiple aspects appropriately:

- a shared vision;
- clear and mutually identified and understood goals and expectations, thereby minimising any hidden agendas;
- an acceptance of diversity and the development of mutual respect and equality;

- a willingness to engage in self-assessment;
- a commitment to openly and effectively communicate, exploring ideas and dilemmas and resolving conflict;
- commitment to the mentoring process from both the mentor and student.

It is indisputable that the establishment and maintenance of an effective working relationship is pivotal in nurturing and assessing the competence of students in health and social care professional practice education. However, as identified by Alho in her case study, these relationships are not always successful.

Establishing effective working relationships – Niina Alho

Critical-care practice arenas are very busy and unpredictable learning environments. For new staff it can be a very daunting experience to commence working in this practice setting, where so many specialities meet and the expectations of staff are high.

In my department we regularly have staff that join us who often have very different practice backgrounds and may have no experience of emergency care. Recently an experienced nurse transferred to our department. This registered nurse had entered a completely new practice environment, facing the anxieties that this move can produce. Initially she appeared to do well and was enthusiastic and the team had realistic expectations of her knowledge and skills relating to critical care nursing. On her arrival she was allocated a mentor who was an experienced practitioner within the practice area and a qualified mentor. The expectation of the organisation was that a formal mentorship relationship would be in place and would include processes such as significant contact between mentor and mentee, structured time for reflection, supernumerary status, and support from other mentors and team members. Initially she enjoyed this supernumerary status; however, on reflection this was for a relatively short period. Ideally the off duty should have been planned around the mentor's and mentee's shifts but due to a number of restraints this did not always occur.

On the shifts that she and her mentor did work together her mentor was often in charge of those shifts, and thus not leaving enough time for mentoring. She was asking other staff for advice and some of those staff expressed to her that she was not learning fast enough and this made her feel uncomfortable. Her initial enthusiasm and confidence appeared to be affected and as a result her motivation gradually diminished. Whilst this was recognised by her mentor and other team members, due to the effects of the organisational constraints on the mentoring relationship it became difficult for the mentor to respond appropriately to the mentee's needs. Rather than this recognition producing more support for the mentee some team members became frustrated and actually withdrew support, as well as implying that she wasn't fitting into the practice area. Hodges (2009) points out that the mentoring relationship can be negatively affected if the expectations and perceptions of mentors and learners are different. It appeared that effective working relationships were not achieved between both the mentor and mentee and the mentee and other team members. Eventually the nurse decided that critical care was not for her. After reflecting on this situation it seemed apparent to me that had appropriate mentoring support been in place there may have been a different outcome.

The mentee in this situation was a registered nurse who was new to a specialist area of practice and therefore perhaps a less formal arrangement would have been of benefit to her. Tracey and Nicholl (2006) have criticised formal mentorship arrangements that are formed as part of the organisational structure, as these don't always foster a common motivation between people and can often lack the fundamental tenets of a mentoring relationship. In addition Petrilli (2011) argues that the connection between the mentor and learner is not always achieved within formal mentorship. More informal mentorship arrangements could have been beneficial to the nurse's learning by emphasising a sense of belonging and a recognition of her value within the team. Wright (2006) points out that instead of appointing a mentor from the department a practice area should consider allowing a mentee to choose their own mentor, and this seems particularly appropriate in this case.

In this case study the lack of support might seem evident. However, it is also important to consider the mentee's role within the relationship. Starcevich and Friend's (2009) study claims that it is important for learners to contribute to the maintenance of the relationship and respond to their mentor's efforts appropriately. Mentoring is not a one-way process and involves a mutuality and reciprocity. Wright (2006) comments that the mentoring relationship is not a relationship if the mentor is not sufficiently engaged with the learner and their learning process. In this scenario the new member of staff required supportive relationships not only from the designated mentor but also from other team members. It is apparent that some members of the team failed to meet this element of mentoring.

This case study highlights the potential benefits of informal mentoring whilst maintaining an appropriate level of structure and facilitation. A recognition of prior knowledge and experience is important in any mentoring

(Continued)

(Continued)

relationship; however, this recognition and value is particularly pertinent when considering the support of a qualified professional. The quality time invested in both students and practitioners new to the area by mentors is essential, but the wider team also needs to actively participate in developing supportive relationships. I can now appreciate the complex skills required to manage this mentorship situation and particularly the importance of facilitating effective relationships amongst the team.

When this is managed effectively the positive benefits include the continued professional development of the mentee; a motivated and committed individual; and enhanced team morale and job satisfaction. Ultimately it can ensure the retention of staff.

Alho's case study demonstrates the potentially devastating consequences of an unsuccessful mentoring relationship.

Ineffective student–mentor relationships

The mentee in the case study above was a registered practitioner and whilst undoubtedly she had a negative experience she will hopefully continue in her chosen profession. For a health or social care student a similar situation may have caused that student to leave their chosen profession prematurely without gaining registration. Alho's case study illustrates explicitly several of the issues already identified, including the role conflict experienced by the mentor: in this case it culminated in the mentor not being able to spend sufficient time with the mentee and an inappropriate balance between formal and informal mentoring. The study also raises the issue of poor mentoring and ineffective student–mentor relationships, and it may be useful for students and mentors to consider ineffective working relationships in the context of belongingness, caring and the influence of power on relationships. Ineffective student–mentor relationships may occur for several reasons, including resource issues and a lack of support for the mentor, professional practitioners who display poor mentoring skills, toxic mentors and students who do not take responsibility for their contribution to the relationship. Alho identified that the mentee needed to develop confidence in a practice area that was new to her. As the mentee did not require summative assessment, the less formal, supportive, aspects of mentorship could have taken precedence in order for the mentee to gain confidence, interact with team members and engage effectively in practice activity. However, the allocated mentor clearly did not have enough time to spend with the mentee and the mentoring was poorly planned. These supportive elements of the mentor role apply equally to students who when deprived of quality support are likely to be disadvantaged. Spouse (2001) identified several features of students who are not befriended appropriately by their mentors:

- students may resort to wandering around trying to find something useful to do;
- students may form clinging relationships with single members of the team;
- students may be forced to constantly seek permission to undertake and practise skills;
- students may miss opportunities to engage in more complex care, ending up repeating tasks that they are already capable of;
- students may lose confidence and withdraw from practice when possible thereby missing further learning opportunities that will result in poor practice reports.

Without the high quality of support inherent within an effective working relationship students are likely to become de-motivated and lose confidence, the results of which will hinder both their personal and professional development. Students report experiences of poor mentoring at some point during their professional education programme (Gray and Smith, 2000). Along with her assertions of what makes a good mentor, Darling (1985) identifies poor mentors as a galaxy of toxic mentors who approach mentoring in a certain negative way. The terms that Darling coined to ascribe to these mentors are as follows:

- Avoiders – these are mentors who are not approachable, available or accessible. They may deliberately make themselves unavailable to a student when that student needs support.
- Dumpers – these are mentors who have a deliberate approach of exposing students to situations that they are not prepared for, and assuming that students will then swim (stay afloat) or sink (and drown). Dumper mentors stand back and do not fulfil their responsibility for students learning.
- Blockers – these mentors consciously refuse to meet students' needs, either by withholding information to hinder their development, declining student requests for help or putting students off until later, and hovering over students, over supervising and preventing their progression in learning.
- Destroyers/criticisers – these mentors aim to destroy students by overtly belittling them in a public arena or subtly but constantly undermining their confidence.

Mentors may not display such extreme traits as identified by Darling (1985); however, they may not possess the level of skills, knowledge and attitudes required by good mentors and will demonstrate a lack of enthusiasm for learning through their practice and behaviours. Gopee (2011) has identified several mentor features that may discourage student learning:

- a disinterest in students and their learning needs;
- a limited application of research utilisation and a reluctance to change practice;
- a hierarchical approach with limited team work;
- a lack of knowledge regarding students' professional education programme;
- a lack of acknowledgement and valuing of students' previous experience and knowledge.

This acknowledgment that not all students experience good mentoring with an effective working relationship poses the question of whether mentorship should be by choice. Currently within nursing there is an expectation that registered nurses, following their period of preceptorship and consolidation, will undertake preparation to become a mentor. Therefore becoming a mentor is not a choice but a requirement that is often reflected in job descriptions. It could be argued that many mentors are relatively inexperienced within their professional practice arena which is not congruent with the notion of the mentor as a wise and experienced person. However, students may benefit from mentors who are closer in years to the experience of undertaking a professional education programme.

Student nurses reported in research undertaken by Gidman et al. (2011) that they felt mentoring should be voluntary, going so far as to suggest that potential mentors should somehow be vetted. These students felt that if mentors did not want to undertake the role then this would have a detrimental effect on students' experience. Over half of the mentors surveyed by Moseley and Davies (2007) agreed that some people are suited to the role and others are not. It is accepted that health and social care professionals have a responsibility and duty to nurture, teach and assess students, thus acting as gatekeepers to their profession, and most mentors view this important role in a positive light. When considering all the benefits to mentors of being a mentor Bray and Nettleton (2007) asserted that the compulsory nature of mentorship did not nullify these benefits. In terms of support for mentors Huybrecht et al. (2011) suggest that high numbers of active mentors in any one area increases the sharing of knowledge and reflection amongst mentors and is one justification for compulsory mentorship.

Mentorship should be an integral part of a suitably experienced health or social care professional's role. However, preparation needs to be robust and mentors should be appropriately supported to ensure they are able to function effectively and avoid the development of unsuccessful relationships.

Belongingness

Health and social care professional practice placements can be viewed as what Wenger (1998) describes as communities of practice. Wenger identifies the necessity of developing and shaping an identity within a community of practice. This is achieved by students through their creation and re-creation of meanings of who they are in these different communities, a process which is vital to a student's identity and learning (Grealish and Ranse, 2009). When students or other learners are new to a practice setting they are likely to experience a degree of stress and anxiety, and it is crucial that they develop effective working relationships with their mentor and other team members if they are to effectively participate peripherally in the community of practice. Lave and Wenger (1999) describe how, with increasing confidence, learners move from a peripheral to a more central position in their community of practice. The nurse in Alho's case study who had moved to a potentially stressful new area of practice was clearly unable to engage in legitimate peripheral participation let alone move to an accepted central position within the community of practice. It is clear from Alho's case study that the nurse mentioned did not have an effective relationship with her mentor and team members who could have facilitated her sense of belongingness, a strong sense of which may have empowered her within that community of practice. Levett-Jones et al. (2007) describe the concept of belongingness as including feelings of a sense of connectedness, fitting in and being involved with, cared for and valued by others. Belongingness has a positive impact on student development in a number of ways:

- it serves to facilitate the appropriate socialisation of students into their chosen profession;
- it serves to increase student motivation;
- it serves to increase students' confidence to question and challenge.

Students reported in research undertaken by Levett-Jones and Lathlean (2008) that a sense of belongingness influenced their motivation and capacity to engage in learning opportunities in practice. These students described how, when they felt accepted and valued by the team, they could concentrate on learning as opposed to being concerned with interpersonal relationships. The nurse in Alho's case study appeared to have been deprived of a sense of belongingness by both her mentor and the team members and was therefore alienated from the team, leading to a loss of confidence and hindered learning. Given that in further research Levett-Jones et al's (2009) students identified that their relationships with staff impacted on their sense of belonging and the quality of their placement and learning, mentors need to recognise their significant role in fostering effective relationships between team members and students.

It is also a key consideration for mentors to achieve a balance in facilitating a student's socialisation into the relevant profession and to foster that student's ability to question and challenge. Professional socialisation is a complex process in which a student will develop the knowledge, skills and attitudes related to their chosen profession, and will internalise the values and norms held by members of that profession (Ousey, 2009). The health and social care professions need their future practitioners to have critical thinking skills in order to function effectively in contemporary health and social care practice as well as innovate and lead. If students feel safe in their working relationships they are more likely to question and challenge as opposed to conforming if they feel alienated. When a student does have a sense of belonging a mentor needs to encourage them to reflect on the practices, behaviours, norms and values they need to adopt as inherent within their socialisation as well as recognising those they should challenge.

Student responsibility

Mentoring is a reciprocal process in which students have a responsibility to contribute to the establishment and maintenance of effective working relationships. Alho recognised this need for mutuality within her case study, highlighting that students need to respond to mentors' efforts. Po-kwan Siu and Sivan (2011) assert that student–mentor relationships develop not just because of mentor attributes, but as a result of student initiative demonstrated through being enquiring and asking questions, actively learning, being good listeners and showing extra effort. It is vital that any conflict between a mentor and a student is resolved; however, given that students are expected to question and challenge, it would be expected for some disagreements to occur within the relationship. Such disagreement can force students and mentors to reflect on situations and facilitate reciprocal learning.

Grater-Nakamura et al. (2010) posit that students have a responsibility to be receptive to their mentors and the learning that the mentoring experience offers, and they outline several aspects of the responsibility students have:

- to openly share concerns, thoughts and ideas with a mentor;
- to be receptive to new ideas and experiences that may diverge from their theoretical classroom experience;
- to consider critically the information and guidance given to them by a mentor;
- to plan their own learning objectives and develop strategies to achieve them;
- to share new experiences and insights with peers;
- to seek out networking and professional development opportunities;
- to be committed to their mentor and the process of mentoring.

Health and social care students should proactively take responsibility for their role within the student–mentor relationship, which will enable them to make valuable contributions to professional practice through the application of their developing knowledge, skills and personal attributes. In order to maximise students' ability to be more responsible and empowered within the practice arena, mentors need to consider the influence of power in relationships. A mentor is in a position of power within the student–mentor relationship, in terms of being key to the facilitation of student learning and development as well as a student's assessor and thus the gatekeeper to that profession. It can be argued that relationships within health and social care organisations tend to be hierarchical in nature and therefore mentors themselves may well be subject to a degree of disempowerment. A misuse of power can lead to the devaluing of a student as a learner and, at worst, a student experiencing bullying or horizontal violence in the professional practice education placement. Beech and Brockbank (1999) assert that if the relationship between the mentor and mentee is too hierarchical then the mentoring process will lack any developmental focus. Every mentor needs to reflect on their attitude and approach towards the mentorship process and ensure that traditional beliefs and the activation of hierarchical behaviours do not impact negatively on relationships with students and their ability to thrive.

Chapter summary

Appropriately skilled mentors, who have the ability to develop and maintain effective relationships, are vital in facilitating health and social care students to achieve their potential. Dynamic, fostering, mutual and power appropriate mentor–student relationships will benefit both parties and will also prove instrumental in students' transition from being novices to becoming competent, appropriately professionally socialised practitioners who are fit to practice. The effect of poor student–mentor relationships can be devastating for students, mentors and the learning organisation. It is imperative that mentors, colleagues, managers, the organisation, lecturers and practice education facilitators from the HEI and the professional regulatory bodies all work collaboratively to ensure that effective working relationships can flourish.

Reflective activity

After reading the chapter take a little time to consider the questions below:

- Which communication and interpersonal skills do you excel at and which ones could you develop further?
- How have you ensured that the students you have mentored have developed a sense of belonging and how did the wider team contribute to this?
- In what ways do you act as a role model to your students?
- What strategies do you use to ensure the power issues between you and your learner are managed?

References

Ali, P. and Panther, W. (2008) 'Professional development and the role of mentorship', *Nursing Standard,* 22 (42): 35–39.

Anderson, L. (2011) 'A learning resource for developing effective mentorship in practice, *Nursing Standard,* 25 (51): 48–56.

Andrews, M. and Wallis, M. (1999) 'Mentorship in nursing: a literature review', *Journal of Advanced Nursing,* 29 (10): 201–207.

Barry, P. (2009) 'A critical analysis of theatre as a learning environment in relation to placement duration', *Education,* 19 (12): 433–435.

Bandura, A. (1977) *Social Learning Theory.* New York: General Learning Press.

Beech, N. and Brockbank, A. (1999) 'Power/knowledge and psychosocial dynamics in mentoring', *Management Learning,* 30 (1): 7–25.

Bray, L. and Nettleton, P. (2007) 'Assessor or mentor? Role confusion in professional education', *Nurse Education Today*, 27: 848–855.

Carlisle, C., Calman, L. and Ibbotson, T. (2009) 'Practice-based learning: the role of practice education facilitators in supporting mentors', *Nurse Education Today*, 29: 715–721.

Carlson, E., Pilhammer, E. and Wann-Hansson (2009) 'Time to precept: supportive and limiting conditions for precepting nurses', *Journal of Advanced Nursing*, 66 (2): 432–441.

Cavanagh, M. (2002) 'Being a mentor'. In J. Canham and J. Bennett (eds), *Mentorship in Community Nursing: Challenges and Opportunities*. Oxford: Blackwell Science.

Claridge, M.T. and Lewis, T. (2005) *Coaching for Effective Learning: A Practical Guide for Teachers in Health and Social Care*. Oxford: Radcliffe Publishing.

Darling, L.A.W. (1984) 'What do nurses want in a mentor?', *Journal of Nursing Administration*, 14 (10): 42–44.

Darling, L.A.W. (1985) 'What to do about toxic mentors?', *Journal of Nursing Administration*, 15 (95): 43–44.

De Shazer, S. (1994) *Words were Originally Magic*. New York: Norton & Co.

Drake, D.B. (2008) 'Reflections on applications of coaching'. In D.B. Drake, D. Brennan and K. Gortz (eds), *The Philosophy and Practice of Coaching*. Chichester: Wiley.

Duffy, K. (2004) *Failing Students: A Qualitative Study of Factors that Influence the Decisions Regarding Assessment of Students' Competence in Practice*. Glasgow: Caledonian University.

Edwards, H., Smith, S., Courtney, M., Finlayson, K. and Chapman, H. (2004) 'Impact of clinical placement location on nursing students' competence and preparedness for practice', *Nurse Education Today*, 24 (4): 248–255.

English National Board for Nursing, Midwifery and Health Visiting/ Department of Health (2001) *Placements in Focus: Guidance for Education in Practice for Health Care Professionals*. London: ENB /DH.

Eps, M., Cooke, M., Creedy, D. and Walker, R. (2006) 'Student evaluations of a year long mentorship program: a qualitative improvement initiative', *Nurse Education Today*, 26: 519–524.

Eraut, M. (1994) *Developing Professional Knowledge and Competence*. London: Falmer.

Fawcett, D. (2002) 'Mentoring: what it is and how to make it work', *AORN Journal*, 75 (5): 950–954.

Fisher, M. and Webb, C. (2008) 'What do midwifery mentors need? Priorities and impact of experience and qualification', *Learning in Health and Social Care*, 8 (1): 33–46.

Foster-Turner, J. (2006) *Coaching and Mentoring in Health and Social Care: The Essentials of Practice for Professionals and Organisations*. Oxford: Radcliffe.

Gidman, J., McIntosh, A., Melling, K. and Smith, D. (2011) 'Student perceptions of support in practice', *Nurse Education in Practice,* 11: 351–355.

Gopee, N. (2011) *Mentoring and Supervision in Healthcare* (2nd edn). London: Sage.

Grater-Nakamura, C., Aquillina-Arnold. J., Keates, K. and Lane, L. (2010) 'Does mentoring play a role in the transition from student to dental hygienist?', *Canadian Journal of Dental Hygiene,* 44 (6): 247–255.

Gray, M. and Smith, L. (2000) 'The qualities of an effective mentor from the student nurse's perspective: findings from a longitudinal qualitative study', *Journal of Advanced Nursing,* 32 (6): 1542–1549.

Grealish, L. and Ranse, K. (2009) 'An exploratory study of first year nursing students' learning in the clinical workplace', *Contemporary Nurse,* 33 (1): 80–92.

Health and Care Professions Council (2012) *Standards of Education and Training*. London: HCPC.

Henwood, S. and Lister, J. (2007) *NLP and Coaching for Healthcare Professionals: Developing Expert Practice*. London: Wiley.

Hodges, B. (2009) 'Factors that can influence mentorship relationships', *Paediatric Nursing,* 21 (6): 32–35.

Huybrecht, S., Loeckx, W., Quaeyhaegens, Y., De Tobel, D. and Mistiaen, W. (2011) 'Mentoring in nursing education: perceived characteristics of mentors and the consequences of mentorship', *Nurse Education Today,* 31: 274–278.

Kim-Berg, I. and Szabo, P. (2005) *Brief Coaching for Lasting Solutions*. New York: Norton.

Kinnell, D. and Hughes, P. (2010) *Mentoring Nursing and Healthcare Students*. London: Sage.

Lave, J. and Wenger. I. (1999) *Situated Learning: Legitimate Peripheral Participation*. Cambridge: Cambridge University Press.

Levett-Jones, T., Lathlean, J., McMillan, M. and Higgins, I. (2007) 'Belongingness: a montage of nursing students' stories of their clinical placement experiences', *Contemporary Nurse,* 24: 162–174.

Levett-Jones, T. and Lathlean, J. (2008) 'Belongingness: a prerequisite for nursing students' clinical learning', *Nurse Education in Practice,* 8: 103–111.

Levett-Jones, T., Lathlean, J., Higgins, I. and McMillan, M. (2009) 'Staff-student relationships and their impact on nursing students' belongingness and learning', *Journal of Advanced Nursing,* 65 (2): 316–324.

Maslow, A. (1987) *Motivation and Personality* (3rd edn). New York: Harper & Row.

Melincavage, S. (2011) 'Student nurses' experiences of anxiety in the clinical setting', *Nurse Education Today*, 31: 785–789.

Morton-Cooper, A. and Palmer, A. (2000) *Mentoring, Preceptorship and Clinical Supervision*. Oxford: Blackwell Science.

Moseley, L. and Davies, M. (2007) 'What do mentors find difficult?', *Journal of Clinical Nursing*, 17: 1627–1634.

Myall, M., Levett-Jones, T. and Lathlean, J. (2008) 'Mentorship in contemporary practice: the experience of nursing students and practice mentors', *Journal of Clinical Nursing*: 1834–1842.

Nursing and Midwifery Council (2008) *Standards to Support Learning and Assessment in Practice* (2nd edn). London: NMC.

O'Connor, J. and Lages, A. (2004) *Coaching with NLP: A Practical Guide to Getting the Best out of Yourself and Others*. London: HarperCollins.

Ousey, K. (2009) 'Socialization of student nurses: the role of the mentor', *Learning in Health and Social Care*, 8 (3): 175–184.

Paice, E., Heard, S. and Moss, F. (2002) 'How important are role models in making good doctors?', *British Medical Journal*, 325 (7366): 707–710.

Petrilli, L. (2011) *Successful Mentoring Relationships: Keys to Success. C-Level Strategies – Visionary Leadership*. Available at www.lisapetrilli. com/2011/02/07/successful-mentoring-relationships-keys-to-success/ (last accessed 2 June 2011).

Phillips, T., Schostak, J. and Tyler, J. (2000) *Practice and Assessment in Nursing and Midwifery: Doing It for Real*. London: ENB.

Po-kwan Siu, G. and Sivan, A. (2011) 'Mentoring experiences of psychiatric nurses: from acquaintance to affirmation', *Nurse Education Today*, 31: 797–802.

Ruch, G. (2012) 'Two halves make a whole: developing integrated critical, analytic and reflective thinking in social work practice and education'. In J. Lishman (ed.), *Social Work Education and Training*. London: Jessica Kingsley.

Sharp, P., Ainslie, T., Hemphill, A., Hobson, S., Merriman, C., Ong, P. and Roche, J. (2006) *Mentoring: A Resource for Those who Facilitate Placement Learning* (2nd edn). Oxford: Oxford Brookes University.

Spouse, J. (2001) 'Bridging theory and practice in the supervisory relationship: a sociocultural perspective', *Journal of Advanced Nursing*, 33 (4): 512–522.

Starcevich, M.M. and Friend, F.L. (2009) Attributes of Effective Mentoring Relationships: Partner Perspective. Center of Coaching and Mentoring. Available at www.coachingandmentoring.com/mentsurvey.htm (last accessed 6 May 2010).

Steinaker, N. and Bell, M. (1979) *The Experiential Taxonomy: A New Approach to Teaching*. New York: New York Academic Press.

Sword, P., Byrne, C., Drummond-Young, M., Harmer, M. and Rush, J. (2002) 'Nursing alumni as student mentors: nurturing professional growth', *Nurse Education Today*, 22: 427–432.

Tennant, M. (2006) *Psychology and Adult Learning*. Oxford: Routledge.

The College of Social Work (2012) *Practice Educator Professional Standards for Social Work*. London: TCSW.

Thorpe, S. and Clifford, J. (2003) *The Coaching Handbook: An Action Kit for Trainers and Managers*. London: Kogan Page.

Tracey, C. and Nicholl, H. (2006) 'Mentoring and networking', *Nursing Management*, 12 (10): 28–32.

Watson, S. (2000) 'The support that mentors receive in the clinical setting', *Nurse Education Today*, 20: 585–592.

Wenger, E. (1998) *Communities of Practice: Learning, Meaning and Identity*. Cambridge: Cambridge University Press.

West, S., Clark, T. and Jasper, M. (eds) (2007) *Enabling Learning in Nursing and Midwifery Practice*. Chichester: Wiley.

Whitmore. J. (2009) *Coaching for Performance* (4th edn). London: Nicholas Brealey.

Wilkes, Z. (2006) 'The student–mentor relationship: a review of the literature', *Nursing Standard*, 20 (37): 42–47.

Williams, P. (2008) 'Life coaching operating systems: its foundations in psychology'. In D.B. Drake, D. Brennan and K. Gortz (eds) *The Philosophy and Practice of Coaching*. Chichester: Wiley and Sons.

Wright, W. (2006) *Mentoring: The Promise of Relational Leadership*. Sparkford: J. H. Haynes & Co.

3 The Facilitation of Learning

Case studies: John McKenzie, Caroline Swayne, Pauline Keenan and Anna Turco

Facilitating a student's learning is one of a mentor's key roles. An accurate assessment of student competence cannot be achieved if a mentor has not first created appropriate learning opportunities. It is these two functions, facilitating learning and the assessment of that learning, that ensure health and social care mentors are able to protect the public and contribute to the creation of safe, effective and proactive new members of their profession. Chapter 5 will discuss in more detail the complex role of assessment in practice settings. In this chapter we will explore some of the key considerations for mentors when facilitating student learning. An understanding of what we actually mean by 'learning' is a useful starting point here and so the chapter will begin by exploring some definitions of learning and discuss how these can be made sense of in a practice setting. The notion of the adult learner is important in pre-qualifying professional programmes and can shed light on appropriate methods of facilitation for mentors. This will also be linked to learning theories and we will explore a number of ways by which we may structure learning. The chapter will end with an examination of the need for mentors to structure an episode of learning in negotiation with learners.

A practice placement should have a start, a middle and an end. Practice learning can sometimes be chaotic and rely on opportunistic learning experiences, and indeed very often these experiences can be most powerful for the student. The chaotic nature of practice learning, however, also means it has to be crafted within an overall structure in order to create some meaning and this is vital when an assessment of competence is required.

Chapter link

How would you define competence? (See Chapter 4 for some hints.)

Chapter learning objectives

By the end of the chapter the reader should be able to:

- summarise definitions of learning;
- critically evaluate and reflect upon the key characteristics of adult learners and the importance of this concept to mentorship;
- deconstruct key learning theories and critically reflect upon the application of these theories in a practice setting;
- critically review the need for a structured approach to the facilitation of practice learning.

What is learning?

Before we can begin to understand how the mentor can facilitate effective learning in their practice setting we need to establish what we mean by 'learning'. Various dialogues have ensued over centuries that have grappled with the concept of learning. Very simply at one end of the continuum is the notion that learning is about knowing, remembering and doing things accurately; at the other end of the continuum is the assumption that learning is more than the sum of what is learnt. Learning can be trans-formative at an individual, organisational and societal level, and so how an individual 'gets there' (process) becomes as important as the end result (outcome). Learning is often understood in terms of a relatively perma-nent change in behaviour which occurs as a result of that learning. Honey and Mumford (1982) suggested that learning has happened when people can demonstrate both new knowledge and new behaviours. Importantly, they also emphasise the significance of thinking about knowledge in terms of insights and realisations as well as facts. So it is necessary for mentors to consider not only what learners do but also how they can demonstrate the value base informing their practice. For practitioners in health and social care these aspects are crucial to the development of professional behaviour. We will examine in much more detail in Chapter 5 some of the difficulties mentors will encounter when attempting to assess these various components. However, before an assessment can take place teaching and learning have to happen and mentors have to facilitate that learning.

Domains of Learning

A useful place to begin is by considering the areas in which learning can happen: these are described as domains of learning and include the cogni-tive domain, the psychomotor domain and the affective domain. The cog-nitive domain includes intellectual abilities and the processing of knowl-edge, the psychomotor domain attends to the acquisition of skills, and the affective domain highlights the emotional aspects of learning, concentrat-ing particularly on values, attitudes and beliefs. Obviously health and social care practice demands competence in all three domains. Indeed, it is extremely difficult to think of any aspect of care that relies on expertise in just one domain. It is useful, however, for mentors to be able to structure specific learning by relating it to these three domains. Bloom (1956) originally developed a system of classifying educational objectives known as the taxonomy of educational objectives. Table 3.1 shows Bloom's description of specific characteristics within each domain and a hierarchy of those characteristics.

This taxonomy can be helpful for mentors when deconstructing aspects of learning and also considering at what level students should perform an activity. If we consider the practice activity of a first contact assessment, students would need to know about the principles of assessment, the

Table 3.1 Domains of learning

Cognitive Knowledge	Affective Attitude	Psychomotor Skills
Recall data	Receive	Imitate
Understand	Respond	Manipulate
Apply	Value	Develop precision
Analyse	Organise	Articulate
Synthesise	Internalise	Naturalise
Evaluate		

purpose of the assessment, diagnostic criteria (or similar), any ethical or legal considerations, and the correct documentation. They may also need to complete some technical procedures (for example, taking a blood pressure or doing a urine test). All of these practice activities will need to be completed in a professional manner that shows care and compassion towards the service user. A mentor would expect very different behaviours from a first-year student from those of a third-year student. The distinguishing features of the performance of the third-year student may be their ability to evaluate multiple sources of information, to conduct procedures in a natural and confident manner, and to demonstrate professional attitudes without thinking about these. These behaviours may need to be considered much more by the first-year student and as such they may feel less natural for that student.

Chapter link

What are the challenges in assessing these domains? (See Chapter 4 for a further discussion.)

The first case study in this chapter looks at the idea of novice and expert behaviours. In it John McKenzie describes his attempts to encourage skilled practitioners to transfer their knowledge and skills to more novice colleagues.

The process of enabling skilled parenting education practitioners to transfer their intuitive skills to more novice colleagues – John McKenzie

He who knows not, and knows not that he knows not, is a fool – shun him.

He who knows not, and knows that he knows not, is ignorant – teach him.

He who knows not, and knows not that he knows, is asleep – wake him.

But he who knows, and knows that he knows, is a wise man – follow him.

(Ancient oriental proverb)

This case study examines the process of mentorship within a voluntary organisation providing services to a statutory provider on a contractual basis, and addresses the issue of transference of skills from experienced practitioners to novices. In an increasingly result-, outcome- and target-led political environment, it is essential that providers of services can demonstrate the effectiveness of interventions to outside scrutiny. My own experience of a workforce drawn from deliberately eclectic backgrounds has meant that high quality delivery of services rests on an organisation's ability to train and develop its staff team. This applies to all aspects of the work of a Children's Centre; however, it is particularly true for parenting education programmes as a key component of the courses is the skill of the practitioner delivering the course (Scott et al., 2006).

The starting premise for the innovation was the belief that there were, within the family-centre team, a number of skilled practitioners in the field of parenting education, and that the most effective way to enhance the skills of the whole team was to harness that experience. The National Academy of Parenting Practitioners identified the core skills of parenting practitioners as encompassing the ability to:

- build and maintain relationships with parents;
- enable parents to reflect on influences on parenting and the parent–child relationship;
- work with parents to meet their children's needs;
- enable parents to develop ways of handling relationships and behaviour that contribute to everyday life with children.

(Continued)

(Continued)

While there were a number of the team who possessed these skills, in many instances, the skills were so embedded and intuitive that the practitioners themselves were unable to recognise them as distinct skills and abilities in line with theories of the four stages of learning/competence:

- Unconscious incompetence – the individual neither understands nor knows how to do something, so the deficit is not recognised and there is no desire to change.
- Conscious incompetence – the individual does not understand or know how to do something; however, the deficit is recognised although not yet addressed.
- Conscious competence – the individual understands or knows how to do something; however, this requires high levels of thought or concentration.
- Unconscious competence – the individual has had so much practice with a skill that it becomes 'second nature' and can be performed easily; however, they may not be able to teach it to others depending on when and how it was learnt.

I wanted to facilitate the teams' sharing and utilisation of these intuitive skills and abilities. I decided to encourage this transference of skills through the use of a mentoring relationship. Figure 3.1 shows how the incorporation of a number of approaches to learning created a framework in which these skills could be transferred from colleague to colleague. Practically, this transference takes place through a system of co-delivery of parenting courses and workshops, with novice practitioners initially observing a more experienced colleague, then co-presenting and finally presenting under the observation of the more experienced colleague. This process is enhanced and supported through regular monthly parenting team meetings which are partly training, partly organisational and partly developmental.

A key aspect of the process was to ensure that the more expert members of the team understood their skills and developed what Baume (2004) describes as a fifth level to the above model and calls 'reflective competence'. This ability to critically analyse and deconstruct one's own skill base was an essential part of their development, particularly in enabling them to transfer that knowledge to others.

Using the exhortation 'If you've got it FLAUNT it', where FLAUNT was a mnemonic for **F**acilitating **L**earning **A**mong **U**nskilled **N**ovice **T**eachers, the team were encouraged to unpick their intuitive abilities and assist others in gaining the confidence and skills to deliver parenting programmes (Figure 3.1).

On reflection this project has highlighted the three-stage process which had to be implemented in order to develop the mentorship of the parenting team. Firstly, there was the establishment of a systemic and organisational ethos that encouraged learning and sharing together and an opportunity to practice. Secondly, there was the implementation of an educative process that introduced and supported the parenting educators into a mentoring role. Thirdly, in order to facilitate a mentoring environment the principles of effective mentorship had to be modelled to, and experienced by, the transformees enabling a true cascade of practice (see Figure 3.1).

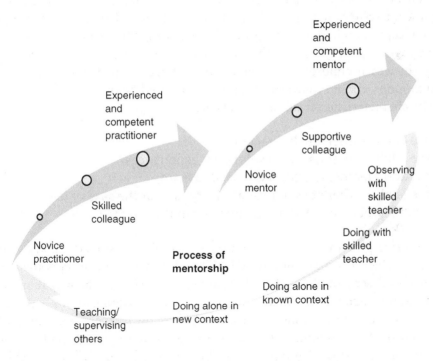

Figure 3.1 Facilitating Learning Among Unskilled Novice Teachers

This case study demonstrates the usefulness of educational theories in constructing a practical programme for developing novice parenting education teachers. McKenzie brings together a number of crucial features in facilitating learning, particularly the concepts of supportive mentorship, the embedding of new practices within daily organisational systems, and an appreciation of the move from novice to expert and back to novice again!

Approaches to learning

Andragogy

There are a number of key writers who have contributed significantly to our understanding of learning. An understanding of these approaches will help mentors to make informed choices about what an appropriate approach should be for a particular learner or learning situation. One of the most significant writers here is Malcolm Knowles (1984, 1990) who developed the concept of andragogy. The principles of andragogy are based on assumptions about the ways in which adults learn. These are contrasted with the ways in which children learn which are defined as 'pedagogy'. Knowles's assumptions about adult learning are summarised below.

The characteristics of adult learners are:

- the adult learner is self-directed;
- the adult learner has had useful prior experiences;
- the adult learner usually has a need to learn;
- the adult learner does not usually learn just for the sake of learning;
- adult learners tend to have an intrinsic motivation to learn.

These principles are important as they inevitably say something about the ways in which learning should be facilitated. If a mentor accepts the characteristics described above then there are implications for the way that mentors should teach adults. An assumption linked to teaching adults is the idea of student-centred learning, with an emphasis on learners becoming self-directed in their learning. This can cause some tension, especially in pre-qualifying professional programmes. Professional bodies will establish the criteria or standards for entry to a profession and these standards will then have to be met. As a result all professional programmes will require assessors to be cognisant of these standards. They will also be required to make sure that the learning is structured to enable learners to successfully meet those standards. However, the process of enabling students to fulfil professional requirements can still reflect the principles of andragogy and student-centred learning. A mentor can negotiate with a student how outcomes can be met, where those outcomes would best be met, and with whom. A criticism of andragogy is the lack of acknowledgement of individual differences in learning: how an individual learns can be a key component in the overall management of a learning experience in practice. Honey and Mumford (1982) have completed a considerable amount of work on learning styles and their Learning Styles Questionnaire can be a useful tool for mentors. Not only will it add some focus to first meetings but it will also allow mentors to consider the most appropriate ways of supporting students. Honey and Mumford suggest there are four learning styles: activists, reflectors, theorists and pragmatists. Kolb (1984) also identified specific learning preferences and these are described as converger, diverger, assimilator and accommodator. Gopee (2011) has since demonstrated the similarities between these different descriptions. A further criticism of andragogy is the observation that not all adult learners will demonstrate the characteristics described by Knowles. As we can see in Harley's case study in Chapter 7, adult learners will not always display the qualities suggested in the literature, and Harley gives a good insight into the challenges faced when working with a 'reluctant learner'.

Learning theories

The study of learning theories can seem a little daunting for mentors, particularly when the practical application of the theories is not made explicit. The case studies in this chapter demonstrate the necessity of having an understanding of learning theories when considering learning in practice. Mentoring students is more than just 'babysitting' them for the period of the placement. Students and mentors must work collaboratively in order to ensure that every student is exposed to appropriate learning opportunities, has an opportunity to reflect upon that learning, and can then demonstrate proficiency via accurate and reliable assessment methods. Understanding learning theories can assist the construction of these activities.

Learning theories can be divided into three distinct approaches which are humanism, cognitivism and behaviourism. We will take a look at each of these in turn and highlight their individual usefulness.

Humanism

The humanist approach places mentors as facilitators of learning and emphasises the importance of the relationship between learners and mentors. Key characteristics of the relationship in a humanist approach are mutual respect and an acceptance that learners will bring with them a whole range of experiences and these should be acknowledged and utilised. The principles of humanism reflect the characteristics of adult learners discussed earlier in this chapter: these take into account the fact that the health and social care learner is an adult who brings with them values, beliefs and experiences that will affect how they learn. They will also have expectations about the learning experience and have other things going on in their life (Rogers, 1996). It is these principles that characterise the humanist approach. There is no single notable theorist associated with humanism; instead a number of key writers (including Knowles) have contributed to the debate.

Phenomenology's philosophical approach can help in our understanding of humanism. This philosophical stance asserts that there is no such thing as reality per se, only each individual's interpretation of reality. This stance places the perception of the individual as central to our understanding of experience. This is significant in relation to adult learners when we consider that they will be driven by concepts of autonomy, empowerment and self-direction (Quinn and Hughes, 2007). Adult learners are active agents in their learning and these qualities and principles should be used by mentors to construct learning activities. Mentors who embrace a humanistic approach will demonstrate definite characteristics as facilitators: they will value and respect students' prior experiences and learning; they will endeavour to negotiate learning and each student will be encouraged to construct their own learning. Effective mentors will also ask for feedback from the learning. Abraham Maslow contended that education should help people to be the best they can be, which is a key underlying assumption of humanistic learning. He believed that education could assist the individual to self-actualise. This links with the work of writers like Mezirow and Friere who articulated the political, transformative nature of education (see Chapter 7 for a further discussion of this).

Chapter link

What are the important qualities and characteristics of an effective mentor? (See Chapter 2 for a further discussion.)

Another notable writer within the humanist approach was Carl Rogers, who while closely linked to psychology and counselling also contributed to theories of learning. Of particular relevance for mentors, Rogers especially described the qualities he felt were necessary in an effective facilitator of learning: these were genuineness (the facilitator should be seen as a real person), trust, acceptance (to create a safe environment) and emphatic understanding (to be able to see the world as a student sees it). Rogers was also keen to emphasise the importance of teaching individuals how to learn. These characteristics can sometimes be seen to be at odds with the mentorship role, and in particular when we consider the introduction of the key role of mentor as assessor where a mentor is required to demonstrate these but also act as a disciplinarian and, ultimately, potentially fail a student's practice. Getting this balance right is perhaps one of the most difficult aspects of a mentor's role.

There are a number of crucial aspects within this approach for mentors to consider. The emphasis on the nature of the relationship between a mentor and mentee is extremely important. However, this approach can also help mentors when considering how to structure practice learning. Encouraging a learner's curiosity and constructing experiences that are both relevant and challenging will help to motivate that individual. Allowing students to 'find out for themselves' will both cultivate their problem-solving skills and again increase their motivation.

Behaviourism

The key components of a behaviourist approach have been challenged by cognitivist and humanist approaches to learning. However, there remain certain aspects in this approach which can be useful for mentors. In some ways adopting a behaviourist approach could seem to be in opposition to the principles of andragogy discussed earlier, but an understanding of the ways in which different approaches to learning can be utilised will only enhance the practice of mentorship. Behaviourists will use the term 'conditioning' to mean learning. There are two cornerstones to the approach and these are classical conditioning and operant conditioning. The concept of classical conditioning was pioneered by Ivan Pavlov. Most health and social care professionals will at some point have grappled with Pavlov's theories and will recall his experiments with salivating dogs. Quite simply he described two types of salivation in his dogs: the first was an unlearned, physiological response to food entering a dog's mouth; the second response, and the one that interested Pavlov, was the dog's reaction when he walked into the laboratory whereupon they would salivate. Pavlov eventually called this conditioning or learnt behaviour. His experiments involved pairing food with a specific sound (a tuning fork). At first the dogs were given food at the same time as the specific noise until eventually, when the food was taken away, they would still salivate at the sound of the tuning fork alone. This became known as a conditioned response. Work by John Watson developed this theory further, as he specifically described how these conditioned responses could be generalised. In his now notorious (and ethically dubious) experiment, he used a nine month-old child (Little Albert) to produce a conditioned fear response when he saw a white rat. From this Watson then observed a generalised response to all white furry objects.

A number of theorists have continued along this path, and in particular it was Skinner who developed the concept of operant conditioning. He argued that human beings could have an effect on the environment they were in and once that effect was noted they could then change the outcome of an interaction. Much of his work was conducted on pigeons and classically the birds would peck randomly at windows until a piece of food was obtained. This random pecking would continue until another piece of food was obtained, until eventually it would cease altogether and pigeons would peck at the window where the food was stored. The key significance of this insight was that the food was now acting as a reinforcer for a behaviour. The pigeons adapted their behaviour and were impacting on the environment. Skinner also went on to describe two different kinds of reinforcers: continuous and intermittent. Continuous reinforcers are given every time a desired behaviour is achieved and intermittent reinforcers are given selectively.

So what does all of this mean for mentors? Behaviourist approaches have been particularly taken to task for ignoring the social context of behaviour and the impact of language and cognitive processes. However, there continues to be a place for behaviourist principles in some aspects of practice learning. In Chapter 2 and Chapter 6 we describe the importance of effective relationships and maintaining an appropriate environment for learning. If we use a behaviourist approach to understand this we can see that a mentor is ensuring that a student associates practice learning with a positive experience. Likewise students who have unpleasant experiences with specific aspects of a role (for instance, when giving an injection or completing a risk assessment) can be helped by their mentor to create new positive associations. A mentor's use of praise can act as a significant reinforcer for appropriate behaviour and help ensure that it continues. However, once a desired behaviour has been achieved intermittent praise is held to be more effective in sustaining that behaviour.

Cognitivism

The cognitivist approach to learning builds on the assumptions articulated by the behaviourist theorists discussed above. The contribution of cognitivist theories is the inclusion of concepts such as memory, perception and thinking. The earlier behaviourist theorists were interested in demonstrating how behaviour could be changed or modified. Cognitivist theories ask questions about the cognitive processes that have a direct effect on learning. As with other learning theories cognitivist theories can be a useful addition to the general toolkit of skills and knowledge available to mentors. This can be especially true when a mentor is keen to use problem-based learning methods and discovery learning. This approach is also useful for mentors when they are considering how to bridge prior knowledge and skills with new knowledge and skills.

Work by David Ausubel highlighted the different types of learning. He was particularly interested in the differences between meaning learning and rote learning and discovery learning and reception learning, and posited in his assimilation theory that most meaningful learning would occur when a learner's individual cognitive structures were allowed to interact with new knowledge. Through this assimilation new cognitive structures would then be formed. This gave rise to Ausubel's other key contribution which was his idea about the use of an advanced organiser at the beginning of a learning episode. An advanced organiser is a link or overview that connects what the learner already knows to what they need to know. If we consider the example of a health visitor who is mentoring a student nurse whose previous placement was a surgical placement, that student may be anxious about their lack of knowledge about health visiting. The mentor in this situation could ask them to talk about how patients were assessed on the ward, about what skills they used, and about how they documented the assessment. The health visitor could then go on to introduce particular aspects of health visiting assessments: in this way, the generic aspects of assessment skills will have already been established. This method of structuring learning has a number of benefits: it can help to increase a learner's confidence; it can help them to identify transferable skills; and it can also flag up good initial assessments.

Jerome Bruner is another theorist who discusses learning using a cognitive approach and examines the merits of discovery learning. This approach can also be of use to mentors as it describes how this discovery can be guided by a mentor using a particular style of questioning to encourage curiosity in a student. This type of approach, if used effectively, can motivate learners to explore aspects of practice in more detail and thereby encourage deeper and more meaningful learning. In addition to a particular questioning style, mentors can also utilise scenarios and case studies to facilitate learning.

Finally, the work of Robert Gagné is important when considering cognitive approaches. Gagné used an information-processing model to explain how people learned. He argued that individuals were affected by a number of categories, all of which were related to learning capability. He described these categories as intellectual skills, cognitive strategies, verbal strategies, motor skills and attitudes. He then went on to explain that these capabilities were affected by internal and external factors. External factors included the way learning was being managed and internal factors were the previously learned capabilities. He then used these concepts to suggest a sequence of instructional events:

- gaining attention;
- sharing objectives;
- emphasising prior learning;
- presenting the stimulus (new learning);
- providing learning guidance;
- eliciting performance;
- providing feedback;
- assessing performance;
- enhancing retention and transfer.

Reflection and experiential learning

In Chapter 7 we consider the nature of learning from experience and the impact this could have on the learning environment. The work of Kolb (1984) is discussed particularly in relation to reflection. Kolb argues there are four distinct learning styles (or preferences) based on a four-stage learning cycle (see Chapter 6). In his theory learning happens when an individual has an experience, is able to reflect on that experience, conceptualise it and then try out something new. This can be summarised as experiencing, reflecting, thinking and acting. This is a useful model for mentors supporting learning in practice as it demonstrates a clear framework for facilitating learning. If we consider the specific example of a learner undertaking a planned discharge then that learner may engage in the process of discharge planning and the mentor would then facilitate reflection on that process. After that they may further encourage the learner to consider the local policy regarding discharge, national initiatives and professional considerations. This learning would then be applied to the next discharge event and the same process would be replicated. The skill of a mentor here is in facilitating a learner to navigate through the various stages of the cycle. They have to encourage the learner to reflect on their actions and learn from both the experience and the reflection. Schön (1991) describes this as reflecting on action, and as learners become more experienced in reflection mentors can begin to encourage them to reflect in action. Schön (1991) describes this as our ability to think about what we are doing whilst we are doing it: this is a specific skill that can distinguish those with experience from those with less experience. The concept of the reflective practitioner is particularly important in pre-qualifying professional programmes and so is also one that mentors should take some time to consider. Argyris and Schön (1974) further added to this discussion by including the concepts of single and double loop learning. Single loop learning can be described as a reactive action that puts right an immediate error or deficit. In this type of learning, behaviour is adjusted to reinstate normality. Argyris and Schön (1974) argued that deeper learning would be evident when double loop learning occurred. Double loop learning is not only a reaction to a problem it also facilitates the questioning of taken-for-granted assumptions supporting the problem. This type of approach can lead to fundamental changes within individuals and organisations as nothing is seen as unquestionable.

The following three case studies bring together some of the key concepts particularly in using reflection to aide learning. However, they also integrate other learning theories within their application. The first of these case studies discusses reflective practice within a new service. Caroline Swayne describes how a new treatment room inspired consideration of the use of reflection in everyday practice.

Chapter link

Can you describe an example of double loop learning from your practice area? (See Chapter 6 for a further discussion.)

Embedding reflective practice in a district nurse-led treatment room – Caroline Swayne

I am a Specialist Practitioner in District Nursing and the clinical lead in a new community treatment room. I have particular expertise in wound care and in the assessment and treatment of leg ulcers and I am always keen to share my expertise with students and colleagues. It was important to me that the new community treatment room would embrace learning and teaching and become an environment in which learning happened.

As the Specialist Practitioner and clinical lead a major part of my role is teaching and mentoring staff and for this I must reflect on my abilities as both a teacher and an expert in order to impart knowledge, skills and attitudes. Knowledge of the range of learning theories was useful in designing the learning ethos of the centre; however, I was particularly interested in the use of reflection in learning.

Knowledge of reflective models is useful for practitioners but not all learners will 'fit' into a reflective model. I was keen to ensure that myself and other practitioners were able both to use reflection within our own practice and facilitate that reflection in others. To ensure this was an explicit part of the learning process I made certain that at the start and end of each teaching session reflection was explicitly discussed.

Donald Schön (1991) is probably regarded as having had the most influence on reflection within nursing practice and he argued that reflection could help professionals to develop their practice. Reflection, both in and on practice, has been actively encouraged for many years. Reflection *in* practice generally refers to the process where the practitioner recognises a new situation and considers aspects of problem solving while still being present in the work or clinical area. Part of the skill of a mentor is to recognise when reflection in action is happening and make it explicit to the learner. I frequently discuss with students and mentors the act of explaining out loud to patients, staff and students. This opportunity allows the observer to understand in much more depth the rationale behind the actions that are taken and the decisions that are made.

Tate (2004) argues that if we impress on students the importance of critical reflection but do not engage in it ourselves then we are simply contradicting our message: our students will neither value it nor believe in it. Role modelling critical reflection and clinical supervision is therefore vital, along with an understanding of the philosophical underpinnings. By engaging in my own critically reflective process, not only will I develop as a teacher, I will also have greater empathy and understanding with my learners and be in a better position to support and guide them on their learning journeys (Tate, 2001).

While much of the teaching within the clinic has been informal and opportunistic some organised, structured teaching sessions have also taken place. At the end of each clinic students and staff are encouraged to discuss that morning's session in a safe and quiet environment: this way I am able to tease out the elements that made it a positive, negative, or just an ordinary experience. This example of reflection *on* action (Schön, 1991) shows the retrospective nature of this type of reflection and the potential power of this type of learning. This activity has led to a recognition of those situations when learning has taken place and crucially when it has not. Reflection and clinical supervision are synonymous because of this perceived value in sharing an experience with a knowledgeable mentor to enhance practice. Feedback from these teaching sessions has proved to be positive and has encouraged both staff and students to review their practice by actively reflecting in and on their daily workload. The activity is also a good chance to role model reflective skills.

The establishment of a new treatment room presented an ideal opportunity to embed reflective activity and learning within the day-to-day running of this treatment area. It has thus enabled mentors and students to participate in reflection in and on action and to consolidate their knowledge and skills acquisition.

Swayne demonstrates the importance of considering learning at the very start of an endeavour in practice. When new services are being commissioned it is vital to consider how a service can facilitate learning in staff, students and service users. It also demonstrates how, in busy practice areas, reflection needs to be embedded within normal practice routines.

In the second case study Pauline Keenan shows once again how getting in early can benefit the delivery of services. In this study she looks at incorporating reflection within an academic programme and describes the implementation of an innovative role within a pre-registration nursing programme. The role of Practice Guide emphasises the necessity of encouraging reflection from the very beginning of a mental health nursing pre-registration programme.

The role of the Practice Guide within a pre-registration mental health nursing programme – Pauline Keenan

The Nursing and Midwifery Council (NMC, 2010) identified the need for mental health student nurses to gain an understanding of the impact their personal values, beliefs and emotions would have on their practice and the emotional impact they would experience through caring for people with mental health problems. The Chief Nursing Officer's Review of Mental Health Nursing (DH, 2006) also called for mental health students to engage in regular clinical supervision to develop reflective thinking as part of their professional practice. The need for mental health nurses to be able to detect and have an understanding of common physical health problems and their effects on mental health was also identified in the Chief Nursing Officer's Review. These considerations initiated a discussion between educators and practice staff who were keen to embed reflection and clinical supervision within the preparation of pre-registration mental-health nursing students. At this stage practice and education worked closely together in a recognition that practice-based learning was central to the pre-registration nursing curricula. The NMC (2010) have specified that half of student learning should be in the practice area.

An initial literature search was undertaken to see what models already existed within nursing and other health and social care professions. A range of roles was discussed in the literature, including Clinical Skills Facilitator, Lecturer Practitioner, Clinical Educator, Practice Educator and Clinical Guide. However, none of these roles combined the specific components identified as being important at the initial planning stage. The role of Practice Guide was created and the following three functions were identified as crucial to the role:

- A formalised facilitation of reflection on practice through structured group supervision.
- The teaching of mental health-specific skills to mental health and adult student nurses.
- The involvement of supporting mentors and practice areas.

The title 'Practice Guide' reflects the emphasis on practice within the role and the need to enable students to navigate through practice experiences.

The local Mental Health Service fully supported this initiative and I was seconded to the role for two days a week from my substantive post of Community Mental Health Nurse where, as a care co-ordinator, I have responsibility for a caseload of adult clients with moderate and severe mental health problems. My cultural historical experience and contemporary knowledge of mental health nursing informs my interventions when supporting the mental health student nurses. Arbon (2004) believes that nurses develop caring and connecting attributes not only because they have experience but also because they have begun to draw upon their experience in a different way. An experienced nurse, according to Arbon (2004), can be conceptualised as a way of being, a positioning of oneself in practice, or an outlook, and this is then connected to an understanding of who they are, what motivates them, and what it is they find fulfilling. This links very well with my main role as Practice Guide which covers the facilitation of structured group supervision sessions with an emphasis on reflection on practice issues. The experience of an expert nurse as Practice Guide can be a powerful resource for learners within a supervisory relationship. Self-awareness is integral to the development of mental health practitioners and clinical supervision allows this to be nurtured in students (Jack and Miller, 2008). I draw on my experience as a mental health practitioner who is equipped with cognitive behavioural therapy skills that are of significant benefit in the facilitation of reflection. My listening and questioning skills enable the students to share experiences and explore various perspectives regarding that experience. Launders and James (2001) suggest that reflection activities guide students towards discovering, exploring and evaluating relationships and help to develop their knowledge, skills and judgement. My hope is that such reflection activities will embed reflection and supervision within student nurses and encourage a new generation of analytical thinkers within our service.

The second component of the role is to facilitate learning regarding mental health-specific skills and to make links between mental-health problems and physical health problems. I do this by playing an active role in teaching fundamental nursing skills in the skills laboratory. These enable both mental health and adult nursing students to make connections between mental health and illness and physical health and illness. This aspect of the role is then taken into the practice setting when adult student nurses participate in mental health practice placements.

(Continued)

(Continued)

The final aspect of my role is the provision of support to mental health placements along with the link lecturer. I am able to provide a link between practice and education and give practical support with issues like documentation and practice placement issues: having neutrality in but also membership of both theory and practice settings improves communication and liaison.

The implementation of this role has been a significant success in a number of ways. The close collaborative relationship between practice and education brought about through this initiative has been of benefit to all stakeholders. The student nurses evaluate the structured supervision sessions positively and it has been a real privilege to witness the development of their critical reflection skills throughout the process. The Practice Guide role works so well because it enables me to support student nurses whilst remaining free from the conflict of assessment and disciplinary responsibilities that the academic and mentor roles inevitably incur. The intended outcome of the role ultimately is to facilitate transformative learning which will support competent therapeutic practice from the registrants of the future.

The role of the Practice Guide emphasises the importance of both reflection and clinical supervision within mental health nursing. Keenan describes the drivers for the implementation of the role and the need for both practice and education to work collaboratively in the establishment of such roles. There is a key message here for mentors, namely that learning doesn't just happen because a learner is exposed to an experience. The facilitator of learning, the mentor, needs to enable the learner to deconstruct that experience and re-create it in a meaningful manner. The Practice Guide role has embedded this formally within a pre-registration programme and mentors should consider ways in which they too can incorporate the facilitation of reflection on practice within their mentorship role. Keenan's example illustrates the benefits of timetabled, structured reflection within a programme.

Finally, our last case study highlights mentors' difficulties in finding time to facilitate reflection while carrying a busy caseload. In many ways it shows the two previous case studies had the advantage of directing services very early on. Anna Turco makes some practical suggestions for mentors to consider when endeavouring to integrate reflection within a normal working day.

Reflecting on a few simple rules for facilitating reflective practice for students within a Drug and Alcohol Team – Anna Turco

I am a Specialist Health Visitor within a Drug and Alcohol Team (DAT). My role is to support parents and mothers-to-be who are substance misusers and as such it is both demanding and fulfilling. There is a great deal of learning available to students who come to our placement area. Very often their experiences on placement will challenge taken-for-granted assumptions and encourage the re-evaluation of personal values. I therefore regularly mentor pre-registration student nurses and student social workers. The placement enables students to develop and broaden their knowledge base and skills and also helps them gain an insight into substance misuse by working with some of the most vulnerable members of society. It also encourages students to explore and develop a wider understanding of the effects of substance misuse, by focusing not only on the impact on children, parents, families and clients who substance misuse, but also on how substance misuse affects all areas of society.

The general aim of all student practice placements is to promote clinical and analytical reasoning and to develop evaluative abilities in those students. The practice placement is a learning environment in which they can develop their goals of integrating theory with the realities of practice and where they can experience and explore the contradictions and conflicts of professional practice. It is within the context of the supervisory relationship between mentor and student that they are encouraged to reflect upon, dissect and understand their experiences during their placement, and where they are encouraged to face the contradictions and inconsistencies that exist within them as practitioners. Johns (2009) describes reflection as a window which allows the practitioner to focus on the self within the context of their own lived experiences. He goes on to argue that this reflection should enable that practitioner to confront, understand and work towards resolving the conflicts and contradictions within practice, and particularly those conflicts that arise between what is desirable and what is actually practised. Therefore, the role of mentor is pivotal in assisting and supporting students to develop and embrace their experiences through the process of reflective practice by focusing on purposeful and selective outcomes for both improving and assessing

(Continued)

(Continued)

their learning and professional practice. Reflective practice is regarded as a key skill for health and social care practitioners and yet the facilitation of reflective skills in others can sometimes be underestimated. This case study describes some of the key skills used to facilitate reflection within my own practice as a mentor. Some of the interventions can seem simplistic; however, it is vital here to unpick exactly what it is that enables students to reflect on their practice.

Often, due to the pressures of our heavy workloads, many health and social care professionals, myself included, can only set aside the time for reflective practice when having clinical, caseload or safeguarding supervision: often our reflection on daily practice is brief, sometimes in passing conversations with our colleagues or even subconsciously about a specific interaction. When mentoring a student I find I am often re-introducing myself to the benefits of reflective practice. In my case this has entailed keeping a reflective journal and prioritising some time for my own reflection during the day. One of the most necessary characteristics of an effective mentor is the ability to role model good practice and this is also true of reflection. A mentor should not preach about reflection if they are not able to demonstrate within their own practice the skills of reflection. Indeed I have personally benefited from listening to feedback from students as they described a practice situation and my part in that interaction. Mentors can use student reflection to stimulate their own reflection on situations.

Finding time to mentor is an issue that is not only prevalent within my own team but across health and social care teams everywhere. The effective facilitation of reflection adds to the pressures of mentoring well. I have had to learn strategies in order to build specific time into my day to facilitate reflection. Within a community team the time between home visits can be invaluable, particularly as the clinical situation has just occurred and is still fresh in the minds of both mentor and student. Ensuring that I consciously reflect on what has just occurred can aid the discussion between mentor and student. This practice has helped me to make certain that reflection on practice becomes an integral part of each placement. A student will often reflect in one of two ways: either 'reflection on action', where reflection takes place after the event and allows the mentor and student to revisit an experience with the intention of exploring and learning from that experience (it is this type of reflection that can be instigated after a home visit or after an important meeting such as a safeguarding meeting); or 'reflection in action', which is often opportunistic and can encourage the student to 'think aloud' as they practise (this type of reflection allows the student and the mentor to be participant observers in practice situations). Of these two 'reflection on action' is often the commonest form of reflection, but understanding the differences between these can assist mentors and students in discovering a range of techniques that can then be used to help develop their professional and personal competences.

The complex nature of much of the work in the team means that utilising a structured, facilitated reflective process can enable students to unpick in some detail the complexities of the encounters they witness. This ensures that their learning is priceless as well as mine! Ultimately students should be able to break down the process of connecting their practical work with their theoretical work. By developing an effective relationship, using open communication and discussion, role modelling reflective skills and identifying appropriate times in the day to reflect, mentors can create an environment in which students will engage in reflection. Ensuring that students are exposed to these processes is an essential mentor role, one that will not only ensure that students maximise their learning but will also provide a strong foundation for each student's professional career pathway.

All four case studies in this chapter emphasise the importance of an understanding of learning theories and particularly the vital role that reflection plays in professional education programmes. A further consideration for mentors is the ways in which these theories are incorporated into their everyday practice. The case studies demonstrate that this takes some thinking about. A clear mentor responsibility is structuring the learning experience. Put simply practice placements should have a clearly defined beginning, middle and end. Ausubel's work and especially his advanced organiser concept emphasise the significance of the beginning of the mentorship relationship. Mentors should invest time at the start of a placement getting to know students, assessing their prior knowledge and experience and starting to make plans for the rest of the placement. Most programme documentation from universities will require a mentor to orientate their student to the practice area and plan how the learning outcomes will be met. A learning plan or contract, negotiated with the student, should be established to ensure that they have every opportunity to meet the required outcomes. At the mid-way point the mentor and mentee should review the learning thus far and make plans for the second half of the placement. It is at this point that failing students may be formally highlighted and specific learning contracts identified. The endpoint of the practice experience will be an evaluation of the learning that has occurred and an evaluation of the mentor and the practice placement. This process is vital in ensuring that learning opportunities are maximised and that any assessment is fair, transparent and meaningful.

Chapter summary

Mentors can be overwhelmed by the sheer weight of theorists and theories associated with learning. However, an understanding of the three main approaches (humanism, cognitivism and behaviourism) can give mentors an insight into the most appropriate methods for facilitating different types of learning. An understanding of learning styles will also allow a mentor to adapt their own facilitation style to meet a student's learning style. The concept of andragogy is crucial in professional pre-qualifying programmes, with its emphasis on student-centred learning and its acknowledgement of prior experience and knowledge. These theories are only useful if they are applied practically and within a structure that supports learning. Learners will require different types and levels of support according to their individual experiences, where they are in their programme and the type of practice placement: all, however, should have a starting point to the experience that looks at what they have brought with them (knowledge, skills, experience) and what they want from the placement and what it can offer. This should be followed by a mid-way 'catch up' that looks at what has been achieved and what is still to be achieved, and establishes where the end point to the placement will come. An effective mentor will be able to take these complex components and integrate them within their professional practice, ensuring that the learner feels the security that is part and parcel of appropriate support and the confidence of a mentor who allows them to manage their own learning.

Reflective activity

After reading the chapter take a little time to consider the questions below:

- How would you describe your facilitation style?
- Which learning approach does it most reflect?

- Think about the last student you supported. Which learning approaches did you use and for what activities?
- Which domains of learning were you concentrating on?
- What do you do to structure the practice experience for students?

References

Arbon, P. (2004) *Understanding Experience in Nursing: Clinical Nursing Issues*. Chichester: Wiley-Blackwell.

Argyris, C. and Schön, D. (1974) *Theory in Practice: Increasing Professional Effectiveness*. San Francisco, CA: Jossey-Bass.

Baume, D. (2004) 'A dynamic theory of organisational knowledge creation', *Organization Science*, 5: 14–37.

Bloom, B.S. (ed.) (1956) *Taxonomy of Education Objectives: Book 1, Cognitive Domain*. New York: Longman.

Department of Health (2006) *From Values to Action: The Chief Nursing Officer's Review of Mental Health Nursing*. London: DH.

Gopee, N. (2011) *Mentoring and Supervision in Healthcare* (2nd edn). London: Sage.

Honey, P. and Mumford, A. (1982) *The Manual of Learning Styles*. Maidenhead: Peter Honey.

Jack, K. and Miller, E. (2008) 'Exploring self-awareness in mental health practice', *Mental Health Practice*, 12 (3): 31–35.

Johns, C. (2009) *Becoming a Reflective Practitioner* (3rd edn). Chichester: Wiley-Blackwell.

Knowles, M.S. (1984) *Andragogy in Action: Applying Modern Principles of Adult Education*. San Francisco, CA: Jossey-Bass.

Knowles, M.S. (1990) *The Adult Learner: A Neglected Species* (4th edn). Houston, TX: Gulf Publishing.

Kolb, D.A. (1984) *Experiential Learning*. Englewood Cliffs, NJ: Prentice-Hall.

Launders, W. and James, B. (2001) 'A comparison of critical thinking skills in standard and non-standard entry diploma students', *Nurse Education Today*, 1: 212–220.

Nursing and Midwifery Council (2010) *Standards for Pre-registration Nursing Education*. London: NMC.

Quinn, F. and Hughes, S. (2007) 'Adult learning theory'. In F. Quinn and S. Hughes (eds), *Quinn's Principles and Practice of Nurse Education* (5th edn). Cheltenham: Nelson Thornes.

Rogers, A. (1996) *Teaching Adults* (2nd edn). Milton Keynes: Open University Press.

Schön, D.A. (1991) *The Reflective Practitioner* (2nd edn). San Francisco, CA: Jossey-Bass.

Scott, S., O'Connor, T. and Futh, A. (2006) *What Makes Parenting Programmes Work in Disadvantaged Areas? The PALS Trial.* York: Joseph Rowntree Foundation.

Tate, S. (2004) 'Using critical reflection as a teaching tool'. In S. Tate and M. Sills, *The Development of Critical Reflection in the Health Professions.* Buckingham: University Press.

4 Assessment and Accountability

Case studies: Karan Jewell, Hillary Gale and Sue Wilson

Assessing practice learning is a vital component within pre-registration health and social care educational programmes that leads to registration as a health or social care professional. The public have a right to expect that qualified health and social care professionals will be safe, competent, caring, and proactive practitioners. The mentors of nursing, health and social care students thus have significant responsibility and accountability for the assessment of students' competence and fitness to practice (Nursing and Midwifery Council [NMC], 2008; Health and Care Professions Council [HCPC], 2012; The College of Social Work [TCSW], 2012). The role of assessor, whilst both complex and challenging, has essential benefits for students, mentors, the learning organisation, health and social care professions, and the public.

This chapter will contextualise assessment within health and social care practice education and will review the why, what, when and how of assessment. It will also examine some of the complexities of assessment, including the validity and reliability of assessment, the balance in assessing the technical rationalist aspects of practice and the personal aspects of practice, and the management of failing students. To enhance their learning in practice pre-registration health and social care students need mentors who are skilled assessors. Students identify good assessors as being fair and consistent, able to facilitate learning opportunities that enable them to be assessed against their set criteria and giving constructive timely feedback. This chapter will consider the skills good assessors possess and suggest strategies that may extend mentors' holistic assessments of students. The need for robust and meaningful assessment in professional practice education cannot be over emphasised if professions are to ensure that future practitioners are able to engage in quality, contemporary, health and social care delivery. The first case study author, Karan Jewell, describes the use of reflection as a means to facilitate assessment. Jewell is a health visitor who mentors both pre- and post-registration students and offers the use of reflection in formative assessment as a meaningful strategy in the context of the multiple demands made of mentors. Health and social care students identify the value of mentors who evaluate their learning in practice in a fair, consistent, and valid manner. These mentors are discussed by students and are attributed as being good mentors who allocate time for assessment and give appropriate and constructive feedback which facilitates students' development and progression. It is vital to consider the higher level skills required for assessing health and social care students and therefore this chapter will examine these in the context of strategies for assessment, feedback and failing students.

The second case study describes the adoption of a broader approach to assessing the competence of registered colleagues. Its author, Hillary Gale, is a biomedical scientist with responsibility for assessing the ongoing competence of colleagues. Gale explores the complexities of assessing competence in attitudes, professionalism and problem-solving ability as opposed to placing an emphasis on assessing tasks. The third case study author, Sue Wilson, is a district nurse team leader and experienced mentor. Wilson shares her ideas on gaining service user feedback to contribute to the appraisal of the team members providing nursing care. This chapter will explore the benefits of service user feedback as part of the assessment of a health and social care student.

Chapter learning outcomes

By the end of the chapter the reader should be able to:

- deconstruct the key features of assessment, including formative and summative assessment within the context of the teaching and learning process;

- critically reflect upon their own assessment skills within the mentorship role and evaluate further strategies in order to develop assessment skills;
- critically evaluate the assessment of competence considering the balance within the assessment of the technical versus the personal aspects of professional practice;
- critically reflect on their skills relating to giving feedback and consider the value of gaining feedback from others, including service users and colleagues.

Defining assessment within health and social care practice

Practice placements within health and social care pre-registration programmes are fundamental to the education of competent practitioners. The achievement of practice competencies is just as vital as academic ability and is assessed as such. The concept of 50 per cent practice and 50 per cent theory is well embedded within pre-registration social worker and nursing programmes, with many other health professional programmes following a similar format. This recognition of the importance of assessed ability in practice is also set to continue, with the new standards for pre-registration nursing education (NMC, 2010) maintaining the equal weighting of assessed practice learning and assessed theory. This national position that is stipulated by the regulatory body ensures that all providers of pre-registration nursing programmes have to reflect this philosophy in a concrete manner. The HCPC's (2012: 10 6.3) standards of education and training, whilst not articulating a definitive 50 per cent practice, 50 per cent theory split, do state 'Professional aspects of practice must be integral to the assessment procedures in both the education setting and practice placement setting'. A review of mentor handbooks reveals that providers of pre-registration health professions programmes have taken the essence of the regulatory bodies' standards and communicated this clearly to mentors. One example of this is a mentor handbook for a BSc (Hons) Podiatry programme produced by the University of Plymouth (2010: 22), which states 'The assessment strategy places equal emphasis on achievements in theory and practice'.

The underpinning concept of the equal value of learning and assessment of this learning in both practice and theory within pre-registration health and social care programmes differs marginally in the clarity of its articulation across regulatory bodies. However, it is evident at both national and local delivery level that it is recognised that mentors of health and social care pre-registration students have a pivotal role in the assessment of those students' professional practice.

Important aspects of assessment

Along with the ultimate aim of safeguarding the public and ensuring fitness to practice at the point of registration, the assessment of health and social care students serves many purposes. These include:

- to provide feedback to students about their progress and areas for improvement, including future learning needs;
- to motivate students;
- to develop students' self-awareness;
- to evaluate the effectiveness of the teaching and learning environment;
- to assess competence;
- to diagnose and make judgements regarding the level of student achievement in practice;
- to develop the mentor's skills in relation to their continuing professional development;
- to maintain the standards of the health and social care professions;
- to assure the public as to the trustworthiness of health and social care provision.

When reviewing the health and social care literature regarding assessment there appears to be significant consensus regarding the purpose and aims of assessment, and these themes are captured in Quinn and Hughes' (2007) enduring and overarching three key aims. They assert that whatever form the assessment takes it should incorporate the following:

- student performance should be assessed against the set criteria of the programme that each student is undertaking;
- assessing students should be seen as an integral aspect of the teaching and learning process and not simply as a means of measuring attainment;
- assessment should encourage students to self-assess and reflect on their learning.

Mentors assessing student practice must also understand the types of assessment and how these translate into day-to-day practice. The two main types of assessment are formative and summative and these should also be considered in relation to continuous and episodic assessment. Formative assessment is diagnostic in nature and is described by Marsh et al. (2005) as being focused on each individual student's learning needs, identifying their strengths and those areas that need development. Therefore formative assessment is concerned not with pass or fail criteria but with helping students to develop towards their achievement of prescribed outcomes. Summative assessment is formal and assesses whether a health and social care student has met the required outcomes/proficiencies at the end point of a placement, a progression point in the case of nursing and the end point of a programme. The result of a summative assessment determines whether a student can progress on the programme, be eligible for the qualification and register as a health or social care professional. While it is imperative that health and social care professions have professionally related outcomes/proficiencies/standards that future practitioners will need to attain, the benefit of formative assessment to student development in mastering their craft cannot be overestimated. The value of formative assessment within the context of each student's day-to-day practice can be considered in terms of its continuous nature and its authenticity.

Professional education has moved towards a greater degree of continuous assessment which Welsh and Swann (2002) describe as an ongoing process throughout the programme that involves sampling a student's practice on a regular basis. This ongoing assessment has a key advantage over episodic assessment: episodic assessment provides a snapshot of student practice whereas continuous assessment will give an overall picture of student performance in practice and take account that a student may not have had so good a day and so this does not accurately reflect their real ability. In addition, continuous assessment can help address another two key concepts that mentors need to consider, these being the reliability and validity of assessment. The reliability of assessment is concerned with the consistency with which the assessment measures what it is designed to measure. Therefore a student's performance should measure at a similar base level each time the same assessment is applied. Validity refers to the extent to which the assessment measures what it has set out to measure. All aspects of the learning outcome need to be assessed in order to ensure the validity of an assessment. These elements of a learning outcome may include ethical, reflective and critical thinking skills, as well as affective, cognitive and psychomotor skills. Within health and social care practice education predictive validity is also a useful application of the concept of validity. Predictive validity is concerned with providing indicators as to the future performance of health and social care students. These indicators are more valid when assessment is continuous as opposed to episodic assessment which occurs infrequently, therefore providing limited indications of a student's future behaviour and performance. Issues relating to the reliability and validity of assessment are difficult for mentors to grapple with considering the dynamic and fluid nature of the practice setting. They will need to take multiple factors into consideration when assessing students, including workload demands, mentor role conflict, environmental conditions, a student's anxiety level, external personal factors, a student's preparation for practice, and the health status of both themselves and students. Wilkinson (1999) explains how assessment reliability is strengthened when students' consistent abilities and achievements are regularly identified by mentors over the whole of students' practice placements. Inconsistent and poor practice clearly needs to be identified and addressed; however, if the student has a strong sense of their good practice this can help them learn from their experiences and keep moving on from not so good practice.

Learning the craft of the practice of social work, nursing or physiotherapy as examples is a complex and challenging process in which regular formative assessment and feeding forward can help students work towards achieving their summative assessments. Another notable feature of formative assessment is its authenticity in relation to the practice setting. Summative assessment in practice may be simulated, or if undertaken in the actual practice area it might still tend to have elements of a 'set up' situation. Allin and Turnock (2007) suggest that formative assessment in the workplace gives students a connectedness to work which motivates learning as they can then see a direct relevance between their learning and assessment. Ongoing formative assessment which is situated in the 'real world' of practice recognises the theory and knowledge that come from practice and that these are constructed in the context of the relevant professional arena. The professional requirement within health and social care for practitioners to be reflective throughout their journey of lifelong learning is firmly embedded. In the following case study Karan Jewell describes how she utilised reflection as a strategy in order to undertake a formative assessment with a junior team member.

Using reflection in a formative assessment – Karan Jewell

This case study will discuss using reflection as part of the assessment process. The concept of reflection is now widely and diversely used (Kember et al., 2001), and, indeed, is a prerequisite for all nurses, midwives and health visitors (NMC, 2005). Reflection can be defined as a way of exploring and evaluating previous experiences and appreciating their impact on the personal self (Williams and Lowes, 2001). I feel that reflection can be used, not only as a way of enhancing our practice, but also as a very useful way of assessing practice.

I am a health visitor who regularly mentors students. As health visitors, we experience a wide range of learners in our practice area. These can include pre-registration student nurses, qualified staff in skill-mix roles (i.e. staff nurses and nursery nurses), newly appointed staff nurses from other disciplines and specialist practitioner students. Amicus (2009: 257) recognises that mentoring can be a stressful role for health visitors, as practitioners are expected to 'straddle two professionalisms (teaching and clinical practice), whilst trying to ensure clinical practice takes place and workload commitments are met'.

I was mentoring a staff nurse from within my skill mix team who was undertaking a degree in community nursing. This degree was unique to our local area, and this qualification would enable him to hold accountability for a small caseload of core (routine) health visiting clients. Often students who come on placement with us are experienced nurses, and are mentors themselves. In practice, I have found this to be useful, as these learners are already used to using reflection within their own practice, and so have an excellent understanding of how we could use reflection when assessing them. However, mentoring colleagues can also have challenges and disadvantages: as Wilkes (2006) argues, friendships are often formed and these can raise concerns that students' achievements may not be a true reflection of their competency as their mentor's assessment may be subjective.

What we did

In contrast to when I mentor pre-registration student nurses, my colleague did not have learning outcomes that would form part of a summative assessment. Instead, we used our local health visiting service staff nurse competencies to continually assess his ability to work at a higher level of

(Continued)

(Continued)

practice, while he was completing his academic qualifications via the local nurse education centre.

Competencies set the performance expectations for professionals working in a field, and the purpose of meeting competencies is to have a competent workforce who will be able to protect the patients and clients they work with. Our local staff nurse competencies have been created by health visitors and managers from the local community nursing service. The assessment process we were using in practice to assess my student's progress in meeting his competencies was purely formative, and therefore I felt that using reflection would be a useful way to assess this.

There are many arguments within the literature that question the reliability of reflection as a method of assessment, as reflection does not lend itself to quantifiable methods and there are varied interpretations of what constitutes a good piece of reflection (Bulman and Schutz, 2008). Price (2005) believes that students do not always appreciate the ways in which mentors use reflection to help them achieve learning goals, and some authors would argue that the process of reflection can be manipulated to meet desired outcomes (Smith and Jack, 2005), which puts its reliability as a tool of assessment into question. Using reflection for assessment can be challenging as mentors and students utilise reflection in so many different and potentially confusing ways (Price, 2005), and so it is essential to always be clear about the ways in which we plan to use reflection to make assessments. With my student, we set aside regular time for reflective discussions about client contacts, and we used role play to mimic nurse prescribing actions, and also to simulate potential challenging situations: we then used reflection to assess how he had acted, what he had felt, and what he had learnt from those situations. I also encouraged my student to write reflective pieces as part of his portfolio of learning; however, I did not assess these personal pieces as I felt these should remain part of his own portfolio of learning and self-assessment.

What we found

Mentors have a clear responsibility to ensure learning is prioritised but this can prove difficult, especially for health visitors who work in the unpredictable arena of safeguarding children. In my practice experience I have previously found that finding the time for reflection and discussions with students is the biggest barrier to overcome. Despite this, it is clear that this time for students to reflect on their practice, either alone or with me, must be prioritised. If this is compromised, then it will have a negative effect on the quality of their reflection, and in turn, a negative effect on the outcome of the assessment.

It has also been suggested that if students know their reflections are to be used as part an assessment, then honesty can be compromised (Bulman and Schutz, 2008), and I believe the best way that mentors can prevent this happening is to build positive, nurturing and, most importantly, trusting relationships with their students from the beginning of their placements. The literature argues that reflection is a difficult process to assess, with some authors stating that it should be used to promote personal insights rather than judge practice efficacy (Price, 2005); however, I believe that reflection is one of the best tools we have to enable us to learn from our practice, and therefore I feel it is very appropriate to use it as part of the assessment process.

Reflection on practice can develop critical thinking, facilitate the application of theory to practice and enhance deeper learning, and, as Juujarvi et al. (2010) point out, it can develop the ethical reasoning and practice of nursing and social work students. Jewell's case study highlights how reflection can be utilised for students' formative assessment.

Formative and summative assessment should not be seen in isolation, but instead as when formative assessment is appropriately linked to summative assessment both can offer positive benefits to learning. A useful distinction between the two forms of assessment is offered by Broadfoot (2007), who describes formative assessment as assessment for learning which has a focus on the learning itself with the main purpose being to contribute to the development of teaching and learning. Summative assessment is an assessment *of* learning rather than *for* learning. Its main purpose is to report development, confirm an ability to progress and provide accountability.

What to assess

Pre-registration programmes across health and social care have the common aim of ensuring that future practitioners who qualify from these programmes are able to practise confidently and competently at the start of their professional careers. Mentors have a responsibility to make professional judgements about student competency. As asserted by West et al. (2007), assessing this competency is a vital aspect of a mentor's role in order to protect the public, gate-keep the professional register, and maintain the credibility and standards of the profession. In social work the General Social Care Council (2011: 3) articulates this by requiring 'evidence of robust mechanisms for the assessment of practice and professional learning outcomes to ensure the supply of confident, competent social workers'. The Nursing and Midwifery Council (2008) include in their Assessment and Accountability Standard for mentors an outcome which states 'mentors must be accountable for confirming that students have met, or not met the NMC competencies in practice'. Mentors need to have an understanding of the nature of competence in order to know what to assess.

Chapter link

Take a look at Chapter 7 for more information on shared competencies in the context of health and social care practice.

Broadly speaking competence is defined as a concept that integrates several domains, including attitudes, skills and knowledge. Further to this, Ilic (2009) suggests that competence also includes a health professional's ability to communicate effectively, work as a member of a team and problem solve. While Yanhua and Watson (2011) argue that definitions of competence remain lacking in consensus they also acknowledge some development in clarification of meaning. The regulatory bodies have much unity in their interpretation of the meaning of competence, commonly referring to it requiring the possession of a combination of skills and attributes. These include the attitudes, values, skills, knowledge and personal attributes required to underpin safe, ethical and quality practice in a defined professional occupation. Given the nature of health and social work, it is inevitable that there are common competencies required by all practitioners working within a range of health and social care professions. Holt et al. (2010) describe a collaborative project that has identified common competencies across the health and social care professions. Those identified by the professional representatives centre around communication, team working and ethical practice. The project team developed competency maps to facilitate an assessment process that would consistently and fairly measure the attainment of common competencies that could be assessed by a mentor from any health and social care profession. This initiative reflects the growing trend towards inter-professional assessment that was recognised by the NMC (2010) in its recent standards for pre-registration nursing education. The standards recognise that a suitably prepared health or social care professional can assess a student nurse summatively at progression point one in year one of the programme. This is a significant move away from the stipulation of due regard (i.e. students can only be assessed by mentors from the same profession that those students are preparing for). Mentors are assisted by each student's professional, programme relevant, assessment documentation which includes the pre-determined proficiency/competency outcomes that need to be achieved. These outcomes should encompass the holistic view of competency; however, different outcomes may emphasise different domains. Therefore a written, prescribed competency statement refers to the integration to a greater or lesser extent of the skills, attitudes and knowledge demonstrated by the student in practice at a set criteria level, including an acknowledgement of the effect of a student's performance on the patient/client and the wider practice context. Health and social care learning outcomes for students encompass the ability to deliver safe and effective patient/client care as a central tenet of the achievement of competence. A mentor will assess a student's competence to practise consistently in different practice situations against written competency statements that utilise formative assessment. In the case study below Hillary Gale describes her application of an eclectic assessment framework in assessing the broad competencies of her biomedical scientist colleagues.

Assessment of the continuing competence of qualified biomedical scientists in the workplace – Hillary Gale

CASE STUDY

I am a Biomedical Scientist working within the Pathology Department of a small general hospital, and part of my job description is that of laboratory training officer for the microbiology laboratory. As such it is my responsibility to ensure that the training needs of all microbiology staff are identified and addressed, and that documentation exists to record their achievement of competence and continued competence in all areas of work.

Biomedical Scientists are registered professionals, governed by the Health and Care Professions Council (HCPC). The HCPC provides a set of standards to which all registered BMSs must work. The Institute of Biomedical Science (IBMS) provides a framework for training and the route to qualification as a Biomedical Scientist is well laid out by the IBMS. A trainee must have already gained an accredited degree, and must then achieve a Certificate of Competence. The certificate is awarded when the

(Continued)

(Continued)

trainee has successfully completed a Registration Portfolio. This document covers all of the standards laid down by the HCPC, and the trainee is requlred to provide evidence that they have achieved each standard. An external assessor then verifies that the portfolio is sufficient. At this point the Biomedical Scientist is placed on the HCPC register.

The Registration Portfolio provides the basic qualification level, but once achieved, the student must then go on to specialise in a single discipline, and to achieve this they must complete a Specialist Portfolio in a single discipline. The achievement of specialist status then follows a similar path to that of registration, with an external verification of the completed portfolio.

Once qualified and placed on the HCPC register a Biomedical Scientist must continue to work to the standards of proficiency they have achieved in qualification, and every two years they must sign a declaration that they continue to do so. Biannually the HCPC audits 5 per cent of Biomedical Scientists to ensure that they are achieving the standards set for proficiency.

It is mandatory for Biomedical Scientists to engage in Continuing Professional Development (CPD) and the IBMS has developed a scheme for doing so. CPD activities include attending lectures and workshops, reading scientific papers and answering questions, and writing essays on set topics, as well as myriad other activities which can be shown to be maintaining and developing participants' knowledge and skills. The CPD scheme stresses the need for reflective learning.

From my point of view as the training officer, while I knew that staff were all registered and participating in CPD I didn't have any documentary evidence of their continued competence, as their CPD evidence was their own personal property. The laboratory in which I work had no in-house structure for the assessment of continued competence, and therefore I wanted to set up a framework for this to take place.

The pathway for the achievement of competence from trainee to specialist scientist is highly developed and the documentation is readily available: an assessment of competence at this level is built into the process. However, the continued assessment of staff competence once qualified is not so clearly defined. There are reasons for this lack of clarity, one being that the IBMS training formula is a competency-based training model. Competency-based training is formulated from the behavioural model of learning, and while this is an appropriate model for many areas of laboratory work, it is less appropriate for more cognitive and affective areas of learning and behaviour such as problem solving, attitudes and professionalism. It is these areas that are likely to be the same areas which qualified staff develop as they progress through their careers and ultimately take on more managerial duties.

At the time that I was trying to develop a system of assessment for qualified staff, the Knowledge and Skills Framework (KSF) part of the Modernisation of Pay Terms and Conditions was being implemented within my hospital. I wondered whether this could act as the in-house assessment, as it was a cyclical review process broadly encompassing all the areas that were covered by the HCPC standards. There have been numerous problems with the implementation of KSF nationally, but many of the recommendations which resulted from reviews of those problems had been included in the local implementation. The KSF worked best in hospitals where there was already a culture of appraisal, and the most important message to come out of reviews of the KSF was that it should be part of an existing appraisal system. I investigated the possibility that KSF could act as my assessment system.

KSF is a cyclical review process. Each member of staff produces a personal development plan (PDP) in conjunction with their manager. In the PDP learning needs are identified and objectives are set and there is a halfway-point meeting to check on progress, and then a review meeting at the end of the year to document and discuss the achievement (or failure) of the objectives. KSF comprises six competencies: communication, personal and people development, health safety and security, service improvement, quality, and equality and diversity. Depending on the level at which a member of staff works (e.g. newly qualified or laboratory manager) they must provide evidence that they are reaching the levels of competency that are appropriate to their jobs in all of the competencies. This evidence must be produced at the end of year review, which takes place in a meeting between the staff member and their manager.

The competencies covered by the KSF are very broad. They provide a platform for the assessment of behaviours, attitudes and problem-solving ability, which the task-oriented and competency-based training schemes do not provide. However, by their very broadness they fail to assess staff's ability to perform day-to-day activities proficiently, namely those tasks which form the minutiae of daily work.

I decided that a complete assessment framework would require elements of both systems, and the documentary evidence, could all be assessed together at the KSF review meeting. Assessing competencies such as the ability to perform procedures correctly, the ability to use equipment correctly and the ability to interpret test results correctly

(Continued)

(Continued)

required documentation that was produced within the laboratory. Assessing competencies such as behaviour, professionalism, management skills and communication could be addressed by collecting evidence in such forms as reflective statements, witness statements and meeting notes. I should point out here that there is no culture of appraisal at my place of work. Where documentation did not exist for tests and procedures within the laboratory I had to produce documents and also find the time to assess staff.

At present my department is approaching the halfway point of the first year of the cyclical process. The thought of having to produce PDPs turned out to be worse than the reality and everyone came away with realistic objectives. All members of staff have been given protected time to achieve their goals, and will be given more in the second half of the year. Most of the staff have already achieved some of their objectives and seem on target to achieve all of these by the time the review comes around. It remains to be seen how the review meetings will go, if, as with the writing of PDPs, the thought is worse than the reality.

Assessing competency in health and social care is clearly a complex and challenging role and Gale highlights how adopting a holistic approach to assessment can facilitate students to provide evidence which will demonstrate their attainment of competence at the required level. Mentors need to guide and facilitate students as to the types of evidence they can utilise to demonstrate their practice achievements. This evidence can include:

- guided reflection with a mentor;
- contributions to patient/client care;
- learning contracts;
- anonomised practice-based documentation, for example, care plans;
- their participation and contribution to team meetings;
- evidence of multi-disciplinary working;
- critical incident analysis;
- feedback from other mentors or team members, patients/clients, and their families and other professionals;
- observations and problem solving relating to practice situations;
- personal reflections of learning.

Competency statements within health and social care tend to use a variety of adaptations of recognised models of levels of learning: these include Benner's (1984) novice to expert and Steinaker and Bell's (1979) levels of learning. These can then assist mentors in offering guidance as to the level expected of students for each year of the programme. For example, in social work students are expected to perform to their competency statements by identifying and understanding in year one, applying, interpreting and analysing in year two, and evaluating and critically reflecting in year three. By approaching assessment in a holistic manner, coupled with knowledge of the students' expected level of attainment, mentors can develop skills and confidence in two of the more difficult aspects of assessment of competence, these being a reductionist approach to assessment and the assessment of failing students. The danger of adopting an emphasis on a technical rationalist approach to assessment is that assessing the personal aspects of students' practice may be limited. The traditional notion of a mentor was that they helped and nurtured the mentee by acting as a friend and advisor. The relationship between mentor and mentee was personal, long term, and whilst it invariably included an element of teaching and learning this was informal. Within the context of current professional education the balance of the role of mentor has changed significantly, with mentors now having to reconcile the supportive elements of the role with those of assessor. Mentors of health and social care students undertake criterion-referenced assessment (where particular skills, behaviours and abilities are assessed against a criterion that must be reached). Jones et al. (2005) assert that one disadvantage of the competency model is that predetermined and potentially narrowly defined performance criteria may limit teaching and learning beyond the instrumental, for example ethical and moral dimensions. A holistic assessment of all three of Bloom's (1956) domains of learning will address any imbalance between the technical versus personal aspects of practice for health and social care professionals. These domains are known to health and social care professionals as:

- the cognitive domain (concerned with the possession and utilisation of empirical information and knowledge);
- the psychomotor domain (concerned with the ability to undertake technical/practical interventions with precision);
- the affective domain (concerned with the ability to demonstrate appropriate attitudes and values relevant to the particular practice situation).

While health and social care mentors are aware of the importance of these three domains for rounded professional development mentors report difficulty in assessing the affective domain. Miller (2010) highlights the tendency to focus on the assessment of the cognitive and psychomotor domains at the expense of the affective domain. It may be perceived by mentors that it is relatively straightforward to challenge and guide students in the cognitive and psychomotor domains with a degree of objectivity. However, they may find it more difficult to challenge students within the more subjective nature of the affective domain. When examining complaints made by patients/clients against health and social care professionals many such complaints are consistent with the affective domain of practice. This may be that a professional's knowledge and practical skills are an expected given, whereas health and social care service users may be more concerned with the professional attributes that are cognisant with the affective domain and are subjected to greater variations in the professionalism of health and social care givers. When considering complaints regarding professional behaviour or the demonstration of poor attitudes, it is vital that mentors effectively tackle assessment in the affective domain. Professional regulatory bodies do provide mentors and students with some guidance relating to the affective domain in the form of standards and codes of conduct. Miller (2010) recommends the setting of specific learning outcomes around attitudes and values (for example, expectations in the way students communicate with patients). These outcomes should be explicitly built into formative assessments alongside the other domains. Mentors can also utilise a range of assessment strategies to ensure holistic assessment, including those identified by Welsh and Swann (2002):

- observation of student practice;
- listening to what others say about students' performance, including judgements regarding the validity of this information;
- discussion (this should be a continuous element of the teaching and learning process and involve discussion and feedback on student practice, including students' own reflections).

Concerns around mentors failing to fail students who do not attain the required competence still exist following Duffy's (2004) key research in this area which identified that some mentors passed students clinical assessments even when there were doubts about their competence. Jervis and Tilki's (2011) study found that some mentors are reluctant to fail students who are not achieving competence in practice. The mentors in this study cited several factors that led them to pass students who were not achieving: these included difficulty in assessing attitudes and their confidence in assessment decisions. Watson et al. (2002) argued that assessors will fail to fail incompetent students unless there is very clear evidence of unsafe practice. This assertion once again appears to suggest a focus on the psychomotor and cognitive domains and a failure to take into account the range of affective attributes required for competence. In terms of accountability a mentors' own competence can be called into question if evidence exists that they passed a student who was incompetent at the time of that assessment. It is therefore vital for mentors to understand the multidimensional nature of competence and ensure an holistic assessment of students. The skilled use of feedback is a further strategy to enhance the quality of assessment.

The importance of feedback

The characteristics of feedback include that it is a dynamic process between mentor and student that has the aim of deconstructing students' practice in order to facilitate learning. Feedback involves mentors' judgements of students' competence in practice, based on evidence gained from a variety of sources, and this can be developmental/corrective or positive/reinforcing. Feedback tends to be mainly based on mentors' observation of student practice and their questioning of this practice. Feedback can be formative or summative, with day-to-day practice situated feedback ensuring that students receive ongoing and timely feedback. Reflection can be a useful mechanism by which both mentor and student can analyse the latter's practice and identify the good aspects of this that can be built upon and any other ways by which to improve practice. Health and social care students consistently cite constructive feedback as being vital to their learning and development in the practice setting. Nursing students in Elcigil and Sari's (2006) study identified that positive and constructive feedback was motivating and should be given throughout nursing practice and not just at the end of a placement. There are several benefits to giving feedback to students as identified by Clynes and Raftery (2008), including a sense of direction which increases confidence and self-esteem, increased motivation, and a sense of being a useful member of the team. As well as ongoing day-to-day opportunistic feedback it is vital that students receive formal feedback at set times throughout their practice placement. Assessment documentation within health and social care advocates and expects that students receive an initial, a midpoint and an endpoint assessment interview in which formal feedback is given. A longer than typical placement (for example, six months/one year) will require more formal points for feedback and assessment. The initial interview should include self-assessment by the student and the formulation of an action plan for learning; the mid-way interview should include feedback in relation to the action plan which might need revising in light of identified areas of practice that may also need development before the end of the placement; the final assessment reviews the action plan and documents the student's progress and achievements in practice. Marsh et al. (2005) suggest that a learning action plan should:

- identify areas for development;
- identify the actions needed to achieve learning outcomes;
- detail how these will be achieved;
- list success criteria to establish how outcomes have been achieved;
- set a date for this achievement.

As well as taking note of the structure of giving feedback mentors need to be mindful of how they give this feedback as it needs to be presented appropriately and with sensitivity. It needs to be unbiased, factually descriptive and specific, and presented with clear examples from practice. Expectations regarding development in particular elements of competence should be made explicit to the student, as should the learning opportunities required to progress towards their achievement of competence. Neary (2000) points out that most students are appreciative of the importance of receiving feedback and value the opportunity to concentrate on identified areas for improvement. When considering the use of feedback in managing failing students Marsh et al. (2005) suggest that mentors have difficulty in failing students with attitude problems particularly when they have passed the practical elements of the programme. Project work by Marsh et al. (2005) offered the following suggestions in relation to students who are not achieving:

- undertake an early exploration and intervention with the student (for example, ask why they appear to lack interest);
- show fairness and avoid making assumptions or jumping to conclusions;
- make a clear articulation of the expectations;
- promptly remove any obstacles to facilitate progress;
- negotiate learning opportunities.

If a student then continues to not achieve a mentor needs to:

- give formal written feedback at an early stage;
- arrange a tripartite meeting with a student, a mentor and a link lecturer from the higher education institution;
- develop an action plan that is agreed to by all parties;
- arrange regular formal mentor and student progress and feedback meetings;
- give the student every opportunity and support to progress;
- recognise that some students need to fail.

Gaining feedback from other mentors and members of the health or social care team working with that student in practice can provide a more complete picture of their practice achievements. This can increase the reliability of assessment, particularly in the affective domain where judgements are seen as more subjective. A further valuable and authentic source of feedback is that gained by service users. The following case study by Sue Wilson outlines her rationale for utilising a system for gaining user feedback in relation to team members.

Service user feedback in staff appraisals – Sue Wilson

CASE STUDY

As part of my role as a team leader in District Nursing, I must carry out yearly appraisals of individual team members as legislated at both a national and local level (National Health Service Plan, NHS, 2001; Department of Health and Social Services [DHSS], 2005). This involves spending time with the individual team member and visiting patients in their homes. From my experience patients will voluntarily start to tell me what they think about particular members of staff.

Transforming Community Services (Department of Health, 2009) speaks about using qualitative patient data in the form of structured questions to improve the service. Within my role I am receiving such qualitative data regarding practitioners on almost a daily basis. However, I am not recording or utilising this rich data in any way. I believe it would be good for both patient and staff morale to employ this information in a positive way.

There is a dearth of randomised controlled trails focusing on this subject as it is very difficult to quantify human feelings and experiences. The nature of nursing and living through experiences with patients naturally leads to a phenomenological approach being taken within nursing literature. It is

(Continued)

(Continued)

qualitative rather than quantitative, information needed when you require patients to verbalise their opinions on nursing staff. These opinions are personal and therefore a subjective viewpoint.

It was difficult to find any articles pertaining to the community and to registered staff. There were some relating to mental health and to pre-registration students and I utilised these studies to heighten both my awareness and my reflective thinking on the theme of patients contributing to the appraisal of staff. There are also government documents which appear to encourage 'user' involvement in the appraisal of staff, both at national and local levels (DHSS, 2005). *Commissioning a Patient Led NHS* (2005) talks about improving public involvement in respect of Primary Care trusts (PCTs) becoming patient led and services being more convenient for patients because they are community-based services. If PCTs were patient and community led then surely that community would want to be involved with all aspects of employing and maintaining the standards of health care workers. The Scottish Commission for the Regulation of Care (2009) is actively encouraging clients who use the service to provide feedback on new staff. They also state that managers will utilise reactions about staff performance from service users as part of the staff appraisal process.

Locally our government DHSS (2005) has gone so far as to establish a milestone by offering its employees training in obtaining the opinions of its customers. However, they do categorically state that the methods used will be qualitative. In a study by Davies and Lunn (2009) exploring patients who were involved in assessing the communication skills of students, the majority commented that they had enjoyed the experience and that it made them feel useful and as if they had something to contribute to the episode of care. Askham and Chisholm (2006) do suggest that patients are given questionnaires, either electronically, by telephone, or on paper. These questionnaires will be anonymous and should be analysed by the employer, and the information then collected will be fed back to the health care professional during their appraisal.

I can see that gaining feedback from patients can be a valuable contribution to staff appraisals. When I embarked on this Learning and Assessment in Professional Education module I had no clear idea on how to go about gaining appropriate information from patients to use in staff appraisals. Using a method similar to that above would maintain the anonymity of patients and ensure their confidentiality. It would also protect individual members of staff who may have had a problem with an individual patient, but should highlight good and not so good points and allow health care professionals the opportunity to reflect on how a patient really feels about the care administered to them.

Wilson's key point regarding the value of health care professionals being able to reflect on their performance in the context of how patients perceive their care can be applied to feedback relating to health and social care students. Feedback from patients/clients can add meaningfulness for students and also provide benefits for the service users contributing to the feedback and assessment process. The philosophy and action of service user involvement in the education of social workers and mental health practitioners has existed for some time (GSCC, 2005; DH, 2006; Mental Health Foundation, 2011) and has more recently being articulated in other areas of health and social care professional education. The NMC (2010) now specifically refer to service user and carer involvement in the assessment process in its standards for education. Despite the articulation of its value Debyser et al. (2011) assert that formal client involvement is still not common practice in mental health nursing. Service user feedback can be incorporated into professional education starting at the point of selection. In Rhodes and Nyawata's (2011) study, service users involved in the interview process for student nurses reported two key themes regarding their desire to be involved: these related to feeling qualified to know what makes a 'good nurse', and therefore wanting to have an input into those who would be caring for them in the future, and identifying that if potential students saw them as people first rather than patients this would improve their attitudes and ultimately make them better nurses. Mentors should be mindful of, in particular, the second theme identified when considering the formative and summative feedback and assessment of the affective domain. Patient/client feedback can contribute to holistic assessment as Redfern et al. (2002) point out assessment hinges on a range of views and recommends the triangulation of witnesses. Research by Debyser et al. (2011) identifies clear benefits to clients, students and mentors. The benefits to clients included raising self-esteem and feeling valued through being listened to and having a say. The benefits to students included encouraging them to be more self-aware and reflect more deeply. Mentors also benefited by gaining a deeper and more refreshing view of their students.

Mentors need to be highly skilled to facilitate feedback from patients and clients. They have to ensure that any risks to patients/clients are avoided, including them feeling under pressure to give positive feedback and the feedback being seen as inferior to that of mentors or other team members. Mentors also need to support both patients/clients and students when discussing the experiences that have informed feedback.

The provision of fair, valid and constructive feedback is of paramount importance in the professional education of health and social care students. There is still some way to go in embedding valuable service user feedback as a widely accepted established contribution to formative and summative student assessment.

Chapter Summary

The importance of robust and meaningful practice assessment of student health and social care professionals is recognised and embedded within literature, regulatory bodies' standards, and health and social care professionals' education curricula. Mentors need to possess a range of highly developed skills in order to be adept at assessing their students, including achieving a balance between assessing the technical and personal aspects of care delivery, having the ability to structure the assessment process effectively, giving timely feedback that includes the triangulation of feedback utilising the views of appropriate others, and managing failing students. Mentors should consider and develop further strategies for assessment, ensuring that any such approaches are student friendly, transparent, objective and reflect students' required competencies. The use of reflection may be one such tool for assessment. The assessment of practice learning whilst challenging is a stimulating aspect of the mentor's role. Being accountable and responsible for students' learning and development via the process of assessment along with safeguarding the profession is highly satisfying for mentors. Having an instrumental role in a student's journey to becoming a competent and compassionate health or social care practitioner who is fit for practice surely increases a mentor's sense of pride in themself, their student and their profession.

Reflective activity

After reading the chapter take a little time to consider the activities below:

- How do you view assessment?
- Are you subject to assessment and if so how do you respond to this assessment?

- Reflect on your current strategies for assessing students and consider ways to extend your skills.
- Consider any potential conflict between your assessing role and your supporting role.
- How do you approach the management of failing students and what support do you seek?

References

Allin, L. and Turnock, C. (2007) *Assessing Student Performance in Work-based Learning: Making practice-based learning work*. Available at www.practicebasedlearning.org (last accessed 2 December 2011).

Amicus CPHVA (2009) *Professional Briefing – Practice Educators: Preparing for New Roles in the New NHS*. Available at www.amicus-cphva.org/default.aspx?page257 (last accessed 16 July 2009).

Askham, J. and Chisholm, A. (2006) *Patient Centred Medical Professionalism: Towards an Agenda for Research and Action*. Oxford: Picker Institute.

Benner, P. (1984) *From Novice to Expert: Promoting Excellence and Power in Clinical Nursing Practice*. Menlo Park, CA: Addison-Wesley.

Bloom, B.S. (1956) *Taxonomy of Educational Objectives, Handbook 1: The Cognitive Domain*. New York: David McKay & Co Inc.

Broadfoot, P. (2007) *An Introduction to Assessment*. London: Continuum.

Bulman, C. and Schutz, S. (2008) *Reflective Practice in Nursing* (4th edn). Oxford: Blackwell.

Clynes, M. and Raftery, S. (2008) 'Feedback: an essential element of student learning in clinical practice', *Nurse Education in Practice*, 8: 405–411.

Davies, C. and Lunn, K. (2009) 'The patient's role in the assessment of students' communication skills', *Nurse Education Today*, 29 (4): 405–412.

Debyser, B., Grypdonck, M., Defloor, T. and Verhaeghe, S. (2011) 'Involvement of inpatient mental health clients in the practical training and assessment of mental health nursing students: can it benefit clients and students?', *Nurse Education Today*, 31: 198–203.

Department of Health (2001) *The NHS Plan: A Plan for Investment, A Plan for Reform*. London: DH.

Department of Health (2005) *Commissioning a Patient-led NHS*. London: DH.

Department of Health (2006) *From Values to Action: The Chief Nursing Officer's Review of Mental Health Nursing*. London: DH.

Department of Health (2009) *Transforming Community Services: Ambition, Action, Achievement*. London: DH.

Department of Health and Social Services (Isle of Man) (2005) *Service Delivery Plan*. Isle of Man: DHSS.

Duffy, K. (2004) *Failing Students: A Qualitative Study of Factors that Influence the Decisions regarding Assessment of Students' Competence in Practice*. Glasgow: Caledonian University.

Elcigil, A. and Sari, H. (2006) 'Students' opinions about and expectations of effective nursing clinical mentors', *Journal of Nursing Education*, 47: 3.

General Social Care Council (2005) *Working Towards Full Participation*. London: General Social Care Council.

General Social Care Council (2011) *Risk Management and Regulation of Social Work Education*. London: General Social Care Council.

Health and Care Professions Council (2012) *Standards of Education and Training*. London: HCPC.

Holt, J., Coates, C., Cotteril, D., Eastburn, S., Laxton, J., Mistry, H. and Young, C. (2010) 'Identifying common competences in health and social care: an example of multi-institutional and inter-professional working', *Nurse Education Today*, 30: 264–270.

Ilic, D. (2009) 'Assessing competency in evidence based practice: strengths and limitations of current tools in practice', *BMC Medical Education*, 9 (53).

Jervis, A. and Tilki, M. (2011) 'Why are nurse mentors failing to fail student nurses who do not meet clinical performance standards?', *British Journal of Nursing*, 20 (9): 582–587.

Jones, M., Nettelton, P. and Smith, L. (2005) 'The mentoring chameleon – a critical analysis of mentors' and mentees' perceptions of the mentoring role in professional education and training programmes for teachers, nurses, midwives and doctors'. Paper presented at the British Educational Research Association Annual Conference, University of Glamorgan, 14–17 September.

Juujarvi, S., Pesso, K. and Myyry, L. (2010) 'Care-based ethical reasoning among first-year nursing and social services students', *Journal of Advanced Nursing*, 67 (2): 418–427.

Kember, D., Jones, A., Loke, A.Y., McKay, J., Sinclair, K., Tse, H., Webb, C., Wong, F.K.Y., Wong, M.W.L. and Yeung, E. (2001) *Reflective Teaching and Learning in the Health Professions*. Oxford: Blackwell Science.

Marsh, S., Cooper, K., Joran, G., Merret, S., Scammel, J. and Clark, V. (2005) *Managing Failing Students in Practice*. Available at www.practice

basedlearning.org/resources/materials/docs (last accessed on 22 February 2012).

Mental Health Foundation (2011) *Service User and Carer Involvement in the National Mental Health Development Unit*. London: Mental Health Foundation.

Miller, C. (2010) 'Literature review: improving and enhancing performance in the affective domain of nursing students – insights from the literature for clinical educators', *Contemporary Nurse*, 35 (1): 2–17.

Neary, M. (2000) *Teaching, Assessing and Evaluation for Clinical Competence*. Cheltenham: Stanley Thornes.

Nursing and Midwifery Council (2005) *The Prep Handbook*. London: NMC.

Nursing and Midwifery Council (2008) *Standards to Support Learning and Assessment in Practice*. London: NMC.

Nursing and Midwifery Council (2010) *Standards for Pre-registration Nursing Education*. London: NMC.

Price, B. (2005) 'Self-assessment and reflection in nurse education', *Nursing Standard*, 19 (9): 33–37.

Quinn, F. and Hughes, S. (2007) *Quinn's Principles and Practice of Nurse Education* (5th edn). Cheltenham: Nelson Thornes.

Redfern, S., Norman, I., Watson, R., Calman, L., Watson, R. and Murrells, T. (2002) 'Assessing competence to practise in nursing: a review of the literature', *Research Papers in Education*, 17 (1): 51–77.

Rhodes, C. and Nyawata, I. (2011) 'Service user and carer involvement in student nurse selection: key stakeholder perspectives', *Nurse Education Today*, 31: 439–443.

Smith, A. and Jack, K. (2005) 'Reflective practice: a meaningful task for students', *Nursing Standard*, 19 (26): 33–37.

Steinaker, N. and Bell, M. (1979) *The Experiential Taxonomy: A New Approach to Teaching*. New York: New York Academic Press.

The College of Social Work (2012) *Practice Educator Professional Standards for Social Work*. London: TCSW.

The Scottish Commission for the Regulation of Care (2009) *Report on the 2008/09 Audit*. Edinburgh: The Scottish Commission for the Regulation of Care.

University of Plymouth (2010) *BSc (Hons) Podiatry Mentor Handbook*. Plymouth: University of Plymouth.

Watson, R., Stimpson, A., Topping, A. and Porock, D. (2002) 'Clinical competence in nursing: a systematic review of the literature', *Journal of Advanced Nursing*, 39 (5): 421–431.

Welsh, I. and Swann, C. (2002) *Partners in Learning: A Guide to Support and Assessment in Nurse Education*. Abingdon: Radcliffe Medical Press.

West, S., Clark, T. and Jasper, M. (eds) (2007) *Enabling Learning in Nursing and Midwifery Practice*. Chichester: Wiley.

Wilkes, Z. (2006) 'The student–mentor relationship: a review of the literature', *Nursing Standard,* 20 (37): 42–47.

Wilkinson, J. (1999) 'A practical guide to assessing nursing students in clinical practice', *British Journal of Community Nursing,* 8 (4): 218–222.

Williams, G.R. and Lowes, L. (2001) 'Reflection: possible strategies to improve its use by qualified staff', *British Journal of Nursing,* 10 (22): 1482–1488.

Yanhua, C. and Watson, R. (2011) 'A review of clinical competence assessment in nursing', *Nurse Education Today,* 31: 832–836.

5 Evaluation of Learning

Case study: Rebecca Bailey-McHale

Quality is integral to the provision of best practice in both higher education and clinical practice. Over the last decade there has been an increasing emphasis across all health and social care professions on the maintenance and improvement of high standards of service provision. This is translated into the development of numerous national service frameworks and best practice guidelines. It is important to understand the relevance of quality within both health and social care practice placements and higher education. Mentorship is deeply embedded within both and hence any review of the measurement of the quality of mentorship would have to take into consideration these meanings and context. There are added difficulties when considering the evaluation of professional education programmes as inevitably the evaluation of these programmes has to include both theory and practice. The significant changes in health and social care practices mean that mentorship takes places in an increasingly complex and politically sensitive context. The political nature of health and social care practice can have an impact on professional programmes. Orme (2012), in her review of the evaluation of social work programmes, argues that high profile cases have had a significant impact on evaluations of social work education and training. The case study by Rebecca Bailey-McHale in this chapter describes an innovation in the evaluation of mentor effectiveness and proposes a more detailed and formal evaluation of individual mentors. Bailey-McHale argues that the complexities of contemporary nursing practice make mentorship a difficult process and so mentors should engage in a much more formalised evaluation of their mentorship skills. She advocates the use of a 360-degree evaluation of mentorship skills based on the work of Darling (1984).

This chapter will deconstruct the concept of evaluation on three levels: firstly, the evaluation of the academic programme; secondly, the evaluation of practice placements; and thirdly, the evaluation of the mentor.

Chapter learning objectives

By the end of the chapter the reader should be able to:

- critically reflect upon the concept of evaluation in professional qualifying programmes;
- deconstruct the mechanisms used for evaluating the academic and practice aspects of a pre-qualifying professional programme;
- critically analyse the evaluation of the individual effectiveness of mentors.

Quality assurance and enhancement mechanisms

Fox (2011) has described two aspects to quality and these are quality enhancement and quality assurance. Quality assurance refers to the reviewing and judgement of defined standards to determine compliance. Quality enhancement leads to service improvement through detailed enquiry. If we consider the relevance of these definitions to mentorship we can see how the mentoring role benefits from a formal quality review. A key component of any quality activity is reviewing or evaluating that activity. Gopee (2011) argues it is essential for mentors to evaluate their mentoring. The concept of evaluation is not unfamiliar to health and social care practitioners as they will continually evaluate the quality of care they give to service users. As discussed earlier, health and social care activity is subject to a number of quality reviews and services are required to demonstrate their effectiveness in a variety of ways. Hutchins (1990) has suggested that within health care quality incorporates four important aspects: safety, adequacy, dependability, and economy. In the standards to support learning and assessment in practice (NMC, 2008) evaluation is included as one of the eight domains. Evaluation within the standards refers not only to the mentor ensuring they evaluate the mentee's learning and the assessment of that learning but also to the mentor needing to 'participate in self and peer evaluation to facilitate personal development, and contribute to the development of others' (NMC, 2008: 20). This notion of evaluation is also evident in the new Practice Educator Professional Standards for Social Work (The College of Social Work [TCSW], 2012), particularly within domain D. Within these standards social workers are directed to 'demonstrate knowledge of current HEI quality assurance systems and ability to liaise and negotiate HEI processes' (TCSW, 2012: 10). These standards also encourage social workers to engage in critical reflection and use feedback from others to evaluate their performance. This is interesting, particularly in relation to the case study within this chapter which addresses the evaluation of nurse mentors. It is clear from the discussion so far that the notion of evaluation is a key aspect of the quality process within higher education institutions and practice placements, and is emphasised by a number of professional bodies, including the NMC (2008) in their eight domains for mentors.

Higher Education quality processes

Within higher education the Higher Education Academy (HEA) and the Quality Assurance Agency (QAA) are the two key quality agencies working with universities in the United Kingdom. The HEA (2008) stipulate that within higher education the purpose of quality is the protection of the public, the maintenance of equity and performance enhancement. Evaluation will take place on a number of levels throughout an academic programme. Programme providers will have systems in place to obtain feedback from students on specific modules that will relate to the student experience in particular. Orme (2012) refers to these as 'smiley face' evaluations and then goes on to differentiate between two types of evaluation: the first she refers to as 'snapshot' evaluations and the second as the 'moving picture' evaluation. The snapshot approach gives a view of a particular professional education programme at a particular point in time; this approach can also incorporate the 'photo album' approach – however, both approaches are retrospective and so provide a static view of that programme. The moving picture approach, as the name suggests, is longitudinal in nature and will demonstrate changes over a specific period in time: it will also usually involve a number of different perspectives, including those of students, academics, employers and professional bodies.

There are a number of evaluation models evident within the literature. Kirkpatrick (1994) developed a four-step model for evaluation with the steps identified as being reactions, learning, behaviour and results. In this model the results from each step will inform the next. The reactions step is similar to what Orme (2012) describes as smiley face evaluation and involves an overall view of what the education was like. Step two (learning) measures what the participants actually learnt in terms of skills, knowledge and values. Step three (behaviour) requires an evaluation of the extent to which the new knowledge is used in practice, and step four (results) measures how the organisation has benefited from the application of this new knowledge. It is interesting to relate this model to mentorship education generally. Later in this chapter we will discuss how mentors remain accountable for their mentorship and the impact that the practice setting can sometimes have on how a mentor actually performs. Kirkpatrick's model would suggest that the last two stages of this process are not considered as fully as the first two when we construct mentor education.

Nationally, the National Student Survey provides a wider picture of student experience across institutions. These types of reviews are used by a number of agencies and individuals in making judgements about both programmes and universities. All pre-qualifying professional programmes are subject to an initial validation process which will reflect the regulations of the university in which the programme will be delivered and the requirements of the professional body endorsing the programme. This process will incorporate the theoretical aspects of the programme in terms of assessment strategy, academic credits and general structure, and will also scrutinise the practice settings and the support available to students within that setting (Quinn and Hughes, 2007). Once a pre-registration nursing programme has achieved validation it is then subject to further reviews by the QAA and the relevant professional body. The QAA will conduct major reviews every four years, auditing the programmes offered by universities, and any number of further reviews by organisations such as the Department of Health, the Health and Care Professions Council and the local strategic health authority can also take place. Quinn and Hughes (2007) suggest that the purpose of these reviews is to assure the public that the standards within professional education programmes are being maintained.

Evaluation of the practice placement

The importance of quality practice placements cannot be over-emphasised. In Chapter 6 we look in more detail at the learning environment and the factors that contribute to an effective learning environment. From a quality perspective the approval and monitoring of the practice setting are integral to the quality mechanisms within professional programmes. It is the joint responsibility of the university and the placement provider to ensure that quality placements are maintained. One of the key factors embedded within professional programmes will be the auditing of practice placements. The professional regulatory bodies will set out standards to ensure placements are reviewed regularly and meet a consistent standard. These audits will usually explicitly describe the accepted standards for placements and also who has responsibility for what. A good example of an audit tool for health care professionals can be found in Scotland. NHS Education for Scotland have produced an audit tool which identifies the key stakeholders within the provision of practice placements (www.nhs.nes.scot.nhs.uk). These stakeholders are students, individuals supporting students such as mentors, practice supervisors, managers and facilitators, and organisations. The audit asks a number of questions of each of these stakeholders, dividing these into two types of statements: firstly, what the person has responsibility for; and secondly, what they can expect. This tool not only clearly identifies the responsibilities incumbent on students, mentors, managers and organisations, but also the support that each of these can expect within their role.

The requirements within social work are also well detailed. The Quality Assurance Framework for Practice Learning (Skills for Care, 2010) gives a detailed explanation of what should be expected in each placement setting. The Skills for Care document also provides an auditing tool for educators, students and academics. This document details six specific areas for consideration, and these are:

- a system for assuring the quality and suitability of a practice placement;
- the allocation of a practice student to that practice placement;
- the commencement of the placement;
- support arrangements, accountability and role clarity;
- the learning and assessment programme;
- evaluation and feedback (Skills for Care, 2010).

The Health and Care Professions Council in their Standards of Education and Training (2012) also include specific guidance in standard five regarding practice placement standards. It is clear that the maintenance of high quality practice placements is an important feature of the overall quality mechanisms of all professional programmes. Mentors are therefore inevitably involved in these quality processes.

Mentor effectiveness

As we can see from the chapter so far, mentors are an integral part of all of these evaluative processes and are often invited to quality events to discuss with professional bodies the structures that are in place to aid their support of learners in the practice setting. However, there is less emphasis on evaluating the continued effectiveness of a mentor. This is arguably a limitation of the stringent quality mechanisms currently in place. As discussed earlier, within nursing there have been attempts to integrate a robust monitoring mechanism for mentors within the mentor standards (NMC, 2008). Work by Duffy (2003) highlighted the need to review the ways in which nurse mentor accountability could be enhanced. These concerns are shared by other professions as well. The Social Work Task Force (2009) recommended a number of changes to social work education, arguing that the initial education and training of social workers was not yet reliable enough in meeting the objectives of the profession. The NMC 2006 standards introduced a range of measures directed at ensuring mentor and placement quality and these were updated in 2008. Nursing mentors have to meet a number of strict criteria which include the completion of a recognised mentor preparation course, attendance at an annual update and meeting the requirements of triennial review which requires mentors to support at least two students within a three-year period (NMC, 2008). The social work standards (TCSW, 2012) also ask practice educators to support at least one social work student within a two-year period. In her case study Rebecca Bailey-McHale argues that the standards for nurses do not go far enough in ensuring quality mentoring. Bailey-McHale accepts that the additions introduced by the NMC undoubtedly increase the notion of mentor accountability particularly within an organisational setting, but argues that it is difficult to see how they have impacted upon the evidencing of mentors' continued competence and skills.

Evidencing quality mentoring – Rebecca Bailey-McHale

As a surgical nurse who is passionate about education and mentorship, I have been driven over the years to seek out experiences and opportunities which would improve my mentoring skills. It has become a concern to me more recently that the student experience in practice may be compromised by the growing pressures that contemporary nursing finds itself under. The role of the nurse is becoming increasingly challenging due to staff shortages, limited resources, greater complexity of patient needs and the increased responsibility that comes from higher student numbers. As the education and mentorship link for my practice area, I also began to examine how as a mentorship team we could ensure that our students and learners could be guaranteed a consistent and effective mentorship experience. It was through student feedback of their practice experience with us that it became apparent that not all students evaluated our area as a beneficial or enriching placement. Further examination of these evaluations led to the discovery that this was not due to a lack of learning opportunities or experiences, but that the issue lay with individual mentors and the skills or indeed the lack of skills they exhibited in facilitating a high quality, consistent learning experience.

Quality is integral to the provision of best practice in both higher education and clinical practice (Fox, 2011). In fact there has been an increasing emphasis on the maintenance and improvement of high standards in both professional practice and academia. The development of numerous national frameworks and best practice clinical guidelines benchmarks minimum standards of care for every service user. Equally, in higher education the Higher Education Academy (HEA) and Quality Assurance Agency (QAA) ensure that educational provision is of a national standard in order to to make certain that service users throughout the United Kingdom are cared for by health and social care professionals who are educated to a high standard. It therefore seems inconsistent with these health and education standards that there are not tighter and more stringent monitoring and evaluative systems in place for those of us who have responsibility for 50 per cent of pre-registration nursing programmes.

Health and social care professionals and their students are used to evaluating their service to ensure the quality of the care delivery and yet there appears to be very few evaluative practices ensuring that mentors remain

(Continued)

(Continued)

fit for purpose. Duffy's (2003) work encouraged the Nursing and Midwifery Council to review how mentor accountability could be enhanced, and as a result they implemented new standards with strict criteria that have to be met by every nursing mentor. While the introduction of compulsory attendance at yearly mentor updates and triennial reviews has increased the notion of mentor accountability, these have done little to ensure that mentors can evidence their continued competence and skill within the eight domains (NMC, 2008).

Following discussions with my managers regarding these issues, I developed a mentor evaluation tool that could be used by individual mentors to enable a thorough evaluation of their mentoring skills. This evaluation could then be used at a triennial review and as a part of the local appraisal system to evidence continued skills and identify further professional development needs. The tool combines Darling's (1984) work regarding the measurement of mentoring potential with the notion of a 360-degree evaluation. Darling's work offers criteria to evidence mentor effectiveness. For the purpose of a triennial review mentors are required to evidence development in the eight NMC domains (2008); however, within this tool Darling's 14 characteristics of an effective mentor are also used to further structure meaningful feedback from stakeholders. The characteristics are listed within the tool with a brief description of how these might relate to the specific mentoring domains. These are:

- role model;
- envisioner;
- energiser;
- investor;
- supporter;
- standard prodder;
- teacher-coach;
- feedback giver;
- eye opener;
- door opener;
- idea bouncer;
- problem solver;
- career counsellor;
- challenger.

Although the Measuring Mentor Potential scale (Darling, 1984) is designed as a self-evaluative tool, it can easily be adapted for use by all stakeholders, thereby ensuring consistency within the evaluation of mentor effectiveness by including mentor characteristics which have been identified and examined in the literature since Darling's work in 1984.

The concept of a 360-degree evaluation is not new within health care provision and education; however, it is currently not linked to the evaluation of mentor effectiveness. For the purpose of this evaluation tool stakeholders will include students, peer mentors, academics and line managers. A key element of the 360-degree evaluation is the incorporation of peer evaluation. Bailey-McHale and Moore (2011) suggest that peer evaluation should be taking place in any location where pre-registration nursing students learn. They go on to argue that this is already the custom and practice within higher education institutions, and peer support and observation specifically enable an individual to critically self-evaluate and, importantly, to identify their own professional development needs. Higgins et al. (2004) argue that when 360-degree feedback is combined with other instruments it becomes a quantifiable and reproducible tool that is an effective evaluation of competence.

The tool is designed to be used by mentors throughout the three years of triennial review and should provide a much more rounded view of mentors' skills and attributes from a number of stakeholders. The evaluation tool is not compulsory; however, the benefits of its use to students, mentors and the organisation are emphasised. The complexities of contemporary nursing practice inevitably impact upon the quality of mentoring, and thus it is essential for mentors to go beyond the mandatory requirements of a triennial review to demonstrate their continued competence and effectiveness. Use of this tool has enabled those mentors who have adopted it to consider in much more detail their professional development requirements. It has also, importantly, highlighted to individual mentors the advanced skills being demonstrated when they mentor effectively, thereby reinforcing the notion of the value of mentoring within professional practice.

Chapter link

Consider what issues may make it difficult for you to fail a student. (Take a look at Chapter 4 on assessment for a further discussion.)

   This case study highlights the challenges faced by nursing mentors when they are mentoring in contemporary practice. Nurses' role (indeed the role of all health and social care professionals) is becoming increasingly complex: mentors face staff shortages, limited resources, an increase in the complexity of patient needs and growing numbers of students to support (Baillee, 1999; Duffy, 2003; Hutchings et al., 2005). These authors argue that these increased pressures have resulted in the compromising of student experiences in placements. Recent literature highlights three key issues for nurse mentors: capacity/time issues, communication issues and relationship issues. These themes were also highlighted in a review of nursing students conducted by the Royal College of Nursing (RCN) (2008). The RCN surveyed 4500 student nurses via an online questionnaire. Students within the survey highlighted the need for improvements in mentorship and communication in placement areas. Seven years after Duffy (2003) suggested that nursing mentors were 'failing to fail' student nurses, Gainsbury (2010) in a study of 2000 mentors replicated Duffy's findings. A significant 37 per cent of mentors (including some sign-off mentors) admitted passing students they knew should have failed. The mentors in this study cited complicated paperwork, a lack of support from their university and their avoidance of the emotional impact of failing individuals as important reasons for not failing students when they had issues regarding their competence.

   Work by Hutchings et al. (2005) and Duffy (2003) highlighted various issues regarding the quality of mentorship and emphasised capacity and time problems. In Duffy's study the mentors highlighted capacity issues as being a key factor in their decision not to fail students in practice. While this work does have some limitations, other research completed since has also highlighted capacity and time issues as having a significant impact on assessment (Lloyd-Jones et al., 2001; Happell, 2008; Lofmark et al., 2008; RCN, 2008). The study by Hutchings et al. (2005) replicated Duffy's findings and both studies also linked length of placement with the ability to assess students accurately. Other work has highlighted the need for mentors to structure learning, to facilitate access to a variety of learning opportunities, to assist with integration into the team, and to demonstrate excellent communication and interpersonal skills. These studies, while specifically related to nursing, are significant because they highlight crucial aspects of a mentor's role. They also highlight potential issues regarding the effectiveness of mentorship programmes and ongoing support mechanisms for mentors. In the case study above Bailey-McHale argues that these skills and attributes should be much more rigorously evaluated, particularly as mentors are under continual pressure in an increasingly complex health and social care setting. As such they should endeavour to build into their practice rigorous and formalised methods for evaluating their competency. Bailey-McHale also suggested the use of Darling's Measuring Mentor Potential scale (MMP) (1984) as a tool to evaluate mentor effectiveness. The MMP is designed as a self-assessment tool; however, as Bailey-McHale has demonstrated it could easily be adapted for use by key stakeholders and provide a robust tool that would offer a 360-degree evaluation of individual mentors.

Chapter summary

Evaluating student learning is a critical aspect of the facilitation of learning and mentors should view the evaluation process as a key part of their role. Indeed evaluations from individual students will probably offer a mentor useful information about their own mentoring skills, the learning environment, and the wider organisation. Mentors, however, will also have a role in much wider evaluation processes: they may play a part in the initial planning of a new programme, be involved in the review of an existing programme, or engage in annual placement evaluations with a lecturer from the university. Mentors are also required to consider the ways in which they can engage in meaningful evaluations of their mentoring skills. The case study above showed that in addition to professional body evaluation requirements mentors should be creative in terms of the ways they go about this.

Reflective activity

Consider the points below relating to evaluation within your own practice environment:

- Discuss with your university link which processes are used to evaluate the programme you support.
- How do you ensure you remain up to date with your mentoring activities?
- What could you do in your practice setting to ensure that mentors are involved in self and peer evaluation?
- Have a look at the Measuring Mentor Potential scale suggested in the case study and evaluate your mentoring skills.

References

Bailey-McHale, J. and Moore, L. (2011) 'Peer support and observation'. In A. McIntosh, J. Gidman and E. Mason-Whitehead (eds), *Key Concepts in Healthcare Education*. London: Sage.

Baillee, L. (1999) 'Preparing adult branch students for their management role as staff nurses: an action research project', *Journal of Nursing Management*, 7: 225–234.

Darling, L. (1984) 'What do nurses want in a mentor?', *Journal of Nursing Administration*, October: 42–44.

Duffy, K. (2003) *Failing Students: A Qualitative Study of Factors that Influence the Decisions Regarding Assessment of Students' Competence in Practice.* Glasgow: Caledonian University & Nursing and Midwifery Council.

Fox, J. (2011) 'Quality assurance and enhancement'. In A. McIntosh, J. Gidman and E. Mason-Whitehead (eds), *Key Concepts in Healthcare Education*. London: Sage.

Gainsbury, S. (2010) 'Mentors passing students despite doubts over ability', *Nursing Times*, 106 (16): 1.

Gopee, N. (2011) *Mentoring and Supervision in Healthcare* (2nd edn). London: Sage.

Happell, B. (2008) 'In search of positive clinical experience', *Mental Health Practice*, 11 (9): 26–31.

Health and Care Professions Council (2012) *Standards of Education and Training*. London: HCPC.

Higgins, R.S.D., Bridges, J., Burke, J.M., O'Donnell, M., Cohen, N. and Wilkes, S. (2004) 'Implementing the ACGME general competencies in a cardiothoracic surgery residency program using a 360-degree feedback', *Annals of Thoracic Surgery*, 77: 12–17.

Higher Education Academy (2008) *Quality Enhancement and Assurance – A Changing Picture?* London: QAA and Higher Education Academy Joint Working Group.

Hutchings, A., Williams, G. and Humphreys, A. (2005) 'Supporting learners in clinical practice: capacity issues', *Journal of Clinical Nursing*, 14: 945–955.

Hutchins, D. (1990) *In Pursuit of Quality: Participative Techniques for Quality Improvement*. London: Pitman.

Kirkpatrick, D.L. (1994) *Evaluating Training Programs*. San Francisco, CA: Berret-Koehler.

Lloyd-Jones, M., Walters, S. and Akehurst, R. (2001) 'The implications of contact with the mentor for pre-registration nursing and midwifery students', *Journal of Advanced Nursing*, 35 (2): 151–160.

Lofmark, A., Hansebo, G., Nelsson, M. and Tornkvist, L. (2008) 'Nursing students' views on learning opportunities in primary health care', *Nursing Standard,* 23 (13): 34–43.

Nursing and Midwifery Council (2006) *Standards to Support Learning and Assessment in Practice.* London: NMC.

Nursing and Midwifery Council (2008) *Standards to Support Learning and Assessment in Practice.* London: NMC.

Orme, J. (2012) 'Evaluation of social work education'. In J. Lishman (ed.), *Social Work Education and Training.* London: Jessica Kingsley.

Quinn, F. and Hughes, S. (2007) *Quinn's Principles and Practice of Nurse Education* (5th edn). Cheltenham: Nelson Thornes.

Royal College of Nursing (2008) *Nursing Our Future: An RCN Study into the Challenges Facing Today's Nursing Students in the UK.* London: RCN.

Skills for Care (2010) *Quality Assurance Framework for Practice Learning (QALP)* (2nd edn). Leeds: Skills for Care.

Social Work Task Force (2009) *Building a Safe, Confident Future: The Final Report of the Social Work Task Force.* London: Department of Children, Schools and Families.

The College of Social Work (2012) *Practice Educator Professional Standards for Social Work.* London: TCSW.

6 Creating an Environment for Learning

Case studies: Susan Dunajewski, Vicky Taylor and Nicola Howard

The provision of an effective learning environment within a health and social care practice setting is essential if meaningful learning is to take place. The challenges faced by practitioners in ensuring that the workplace is a suitable place to learn are considerable; however, the benefits to learners and ultimately to the practice area can be significant.

This chapter will review the concept of the learning environment in the context of health and social care practice education. It will also define what is meant by the learning environment and place this within the context of a learning organisation. The important aspects of learning in this type of environment will be explored from the point of view of students, mentors and the organisation. The first case study writer, Susan Dunajewski, describes how practice can be enhanced by incorporating a reflective framework within the structure of a health visiting team meeting. Dunajewski is a health visitor team leader and describes her attempts to utilise more effectively the formal learning undertaken by members of the health visiting team. The second case study highlights the necessity of providing relevant learning opportunities. Its author, Vicky Taylor, describes the tensions within a school nursing team in providing meaningful learning for student nurses and goes on to demonstrate the ways in which these tensions were resolved. Some practice placements will have a reputation for being learner friendly and a good place to learn; therefore it is imperative to deconstruct what it is about this type of environment that makes it a positive placement; the final part of this chapter will thus attempt to unpick the characteristics of an effective learning environment in a health and social care practice setting. The third case study author, Nicola Howard, a community mental health practitioner, shares her experience of preparing a multi-professional community mental health team for their first student mental health nurses. Howard details the key factors contributing to the successful establishment of the community mental health team as an effective learning environment.

Chapter learning objectives

By the end of the chapter the reader should be able to:

- critically evaluate definitions of 'the learning environment';
- summarise the important aspects of an effective learning environment;
- deconstruct the notion of time for reflection within the learning environment;
- critically analyse the key characteristics of an effective learning environment.

Defining the learning environment

The environment in which learning takes place will inevitably have an effect on the quality of that learning. McIntosh (2011) points out that many of the key features associated with an effective academic learning environment are also relevant when considering the practice setting. However, practice settings do have specific challenges associated with the facilitation of learning. Recent nursing literature has suggested that supporting students in contemporary placements is challenging (Baillee, 1999; Duffy, 2003; Hutchings et al., 2005). These authors suggest that meeting the needs of growing numbers of health and social care students, staff shortages, the increased complexity of patient needs and an uncertain political context have resulted in student experiences being compromised within placements. Definitions of the practice learning environment are also complex as health and social care students participate in a diverse range of learning environments. This has led many to describe the learning environment as any place in which learning occurs; this could include the classroom, a ward, a community team, their mentor's car or a service user's home (the list is endless). However broad or specific we may wish to define the learning environment, the crucial notion embraced by health and social care pre-qualifying programmes is that learners need to learn in the real world and in order to do this they need to be supported by competent professionals. Many health and social care programmes require students to spend at least half of their programme within the practice setting. This makes mentors in practice settings vitally important for the establishment of professional standards, for the enculturation of students within their chosen practice, and ultimately as gate-keepers for entry into their profession.

Chapter link

List the key characteristics of an effective mentor. (Revisit Chapter 2 for some ideas.)

Important aspects of the learning environment

Relationships

Learners' perceptions of the quality of an environment seem to be crucial and very often this is judged largely on mentor quality. In their work exploring what makes a supportive learning environment, Henderson et al. (2009) suggest it is the quality of the interaction between practitioner and learner that will directly influence the latter's perceptions of the environment and will ultimately impact on their learning. Chapter 2 looks in much more detail at the importance of the nature of the relationship between a mentor and mentee. However, this relationship is also important within the context of the learning environment as it will determine the ways in which a learner engages with practice. Practice is the place in which learners will make sense of their professional knowledge, and the place in which new skills, behaviours and attitudes can be tried out. In this environment a mentor will be the expert practitioner who is able to create the conditions in which these things can happen. Therefore the mentor as expert will role model skills and knowledge and scaffold learning throughout the practice placement. The characteristics of an effective mentor that are discussed in Chapter 2 are essential prerequisites for the facilitation of this type of learning. Patricia Benner (1984), in her work describing the journey from novice to expert in nursing, describes three key benefits of learning in practice. The first element is the interactive and complex nature of practice, the demonstration that effective practice does not rely solely on theoretical knowledge. Practice learning demands an awareness of the interactive nature of theory and real life. The second important aspect of practice learning is the development of perceptual awareness, the notion of intuition or intuitive practice. Intuitive practice requires an exposure to practice situations and develops over time with increased knowledge and experience. O'Connor (2001: 48) describes this concept as 'not guessing or feeling, it is a deep knowing, and a necessary element of expert practice'. Learners will benefit from the mentor 'thinking out loud' in order to demonstrate how difficult decisions are made. The third element described by Benner (1984) is the need for learners to see how practice is prioritised. Expert practitioners will know what needs to be done and will prioritise care needs accordingly.

Work by Price (2003) is useful in describing the progression of the relationship between mentor and mentee. Price suggests that regardless of the environment a mentor–mentee relationship goes through four distinct stages. The first stage is described as the 'strangers' phase in which both parties will spend time getting to know each other. The second stage is the 'explorer' or the getting to know each other phase, and particularly getting to know the ways in which learning will be facilitated. The third stage is the 'companions' stage, where the mentor and mentee will establish their relationship and work together to ensure learning happens. In the fourth stage the mentor and mentee become 'network associates', in that the placement will end but their communication may continue.

Chapter link

How do you facilitate reflection with your learners? (See Chapter 3 for a further discussion on reflection.)

Reflection

Chapter 3 discussed the ways in which learning can be facilitated and reviewed a number of learning theories. The application of these learning theories is important when we consider learning in the practice setting. The notion of learning from experience is significant as health and social care students are placed within the context of a practice setting and expected to learn. The ways in which that learning can be facilitated are key considerations. A vital aspect of any practice setting will be the extent to which time can be allocated for reflecting on experiences within the placement. The assumption here is that students are active constructors of knowledge and as such they are expected to engage and interact within the practice setting. Eraut (2004) describes four work activities that can help students to learn. These are:

- participating in group activities;
- working alongside others;
- tackling challenging tasks;
- working with service users.

The notion of learning from experience is important here. One of the key aspects of a positive learning environment will be the degree to which a student has a range of learning opportunities and the extent to which they are encouraged to reflect on those learning opportunities. A number of key theorists have explored the concept of learning from experience. As far back as the 1930s John Dewey (1938) argued that learning happens from experience when it is recognised that the experience has continuity and interaction. These two concepts suggest that learning never happens in isolation; rather it occurs in relation to previous experience and there must be an interaction between the person and the environment. Further work by Kolb (1984) and Schön (1983) also highlighted the importance of reflection when learning from experience. Schön (1983) introduced the idea of reflecting on action and in action: reflecting on action suggests that reflection can happen after an event and reflection in action suggests that practitioners can critically review their behaviours and values while action occurs. Kolb (1984) noted that in order for learning to happen learners should be encouraged to reflect on a concrete experience and extract meaning from that experience (see Figure 6.1).

A further important element of this is the work of Mezirow (2000) who suggests that transformative learning happens when an individual is able to critically reflect on their taken-for-granted assumptions about the world. This type of critical reflection can potentially produce transformations in

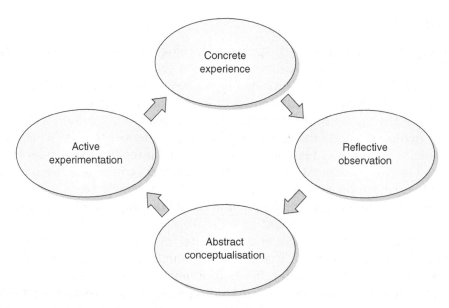

Figure 6.1 Kolb's Experiential Learning Cycle

habits of mind. A key concept particularly when health and social care professions are actively engaging in values-based practice and their own personal values may be challenged by their experiences in practice. The role of mentors is to create learning opportunities within the environment that challenge students' taken-for-granted assumptions and to then support those students in creating new understanding from the experience. The concept of reflecting within the practice setting is a crucial aspect of professional education programmes. It is, however, essential that in order to enable this a mentor is able to both reflect on their own practice and have the necessary skills to facilitate reflection in others. In the case study below Susan Dunajewski describes the attempts made within a health visiting team to embed reflective practice within that team.

Reflection in a health visiting team – Susan Dunajewski

I am a team leader in a health visiting team. I am fortunate to have the support of managers in providing team members with good opportunities for learning both formal and informal. However, I noticed that myself and my

(Continued)

CASE STUDY

(Continued)

colleagues were not always applying learning to practice, or cascading information learned in education and training courses to others in the team. Not only did this result in lost learning opportunities for post-registration nurses but it also had the potential to impact on pre-registration student nurses in their practice placement. Part of my role as team leader is to provide mentorship and enable learning in the practice environment. In order to enhance my role as team leader and mentor I intended to consider how formal learning undertaken by health practitioners could be utilised more effectively, both on an individual level and by the whole team. I believed this would improve both individual and team learning as well as positively influence service provision and so ultimately improve client care. It is an expectation that nurses will engage in lifelong learning and continuous professional development. The aim of this lifelong learning is to enable professionals to expand and fulfil their potential. Nursing has increasingly emphasised the importance of continuous professional development and a requirement for evidence-based practice is a central theme in learning and assessment in practice (Nursing and Midwifery Council [NMC], 2008).

A definition of the clinical learning environment is not that straightforward as whilst it involves material resources which can easily be listed it also involves learning opportunities and experiences, staff members and the wider organisation. I became interested in the idea of transformational learning which involves a more reflective and critical approach to practice, being more open to the perspectives of others, and being less defensive and more accepting of new ideas. This makes it essential to establish an environment in which trust and care are facilitated and sensitive relationships amongst learners are developed. However, as adult learners the rest of the team had to take responsibility themselves for constructing and creating the conditions for transformative learning to occur.

Learning can be made difficult by conflicting demands, with time being used to its full capacity and clinical time taking priority (Clarke and Copeland, 2003). Time pressures prevent not only informal discussion and opportunities to learn from the experiences of others but also the chance for effective reflection. Reflection is a natural part of human life but for professionals structured reflection can provide a framework within which strengths and weaknesses can be examined and strategies for improvement identified. In my experience most practitioners want to provide the best care they can and most managers want to support their staff to achieve this, yet despite these ideals learning opportunities which would improve patient care and health outcomes are often lost because of time constraints and barriers to reflection in the workplace. It was my observation that reflection on practice was happening but often on a superficial level and without the whole reflective cycle being completed; the most essential part ('What would I do differently next time?') was often missing.

There is support for the use of groups and group discussion to facilitate reflective practice and there is evidence that groups can be an effective way of promoting reflective practice (Graham, 1995); however, health practitioners have to be willing to expose themselves to the judgement of others in order for group reflection to be successful. The current culture in which health practitioners work can impose a barrier to reflection. Fear of criticism and judgement can prevent participation in group discussions. A lack of commitment or resistance to shared learning by group members can also significantly impact on the learning opportunities of others. I was aware that it was important for me to consider such potential conflicts and tensions within my own team. Conflicts can have potentially damaging consequences, such as the destruction of initiatives, a loss of team spirit and the desire to work towards common goals, and the cause of hostile and disruptive behaviour. It was therefore important to introduce the benefits of group reflection to the team. I had discussions with team members about my own learning and shared significant literature with them. It was my hope that this approach would generate curiosity and start to create a shared vision, thus fostering a genuine commitment and enrolment rather than mere compliance.

Weekly team meetings were introduced to enable a sharing of information and group reflection. This has improved learning within the team and interestingly has also led to the team identifying areas of learning need. Initially the team reflection felt threatening, but as this progressed and trust and confidence in other team members developed, the benefits of group reflection have actually become a motivating factor within the team. As ever, time pressures have inevitably had an impact on some meetings, with all the team members not always being able to attend and some meetings being cancelled due to the team's workload commitments. However, the process of engaging in structured reflection has undoubtedly helped members to think more deeply about their own practice and consider ways in which they can facilitate reflection in others.

Dunajewski's case study has a number of key points for mentors to consider; for example, she clearly identifies the influence of the team leader or manager within a learning environment. Very often it is the leader of a team who will create the necessary climate for learning to happen. Her case study also demonstrates the need for a clear vision and managers' commitment to investing time and resources into this type of activity. Dunajewski describes the positive effect this has had on team members and so, ultimately, on clients. A further, perhaps more subtle, feature of this case study is the potential fear and tension that reflection can create. This doesn't just apply to team reflection but also to individual reflection. Mentors should be mindful of this when they facilitate reflection in learners.

Learning opportunities

However good the relationship is between a mentor and mentee, and however much a student is encouraged to reflect on their experiences, a placement needs to provide appropriate learning opportunities to ensure that a student can meet the outcomes of their programme. These learning opportunities will include direct contact with users of services and engaging with a wide range of other professional groups. The inter-professional nature of contemporary health and social care practice is evident in pre-qualifying programmes and reflected in practice areas. An effective learning environment will take into account the range of professionals involved in the care of a service user and ensure that students have access to these professionals. In the second case study below Vicky Taylor describes her concerns regarding the use of school nursing placements for adult student nurses and discusses the relevance of this experience for mental health student nurses. At the time the 'due regard' requirements of the NMC (2008) made it difficult to accommodate mental health students in school nursing teams as the majority of school nurses were registered adult nurses.

CASE STUDY

The school nursing team as an effective learning environment – Vicky Taylor

The role of the Specialist Community Public Health Nurse (SCPHN) is evolving and this is certainly the case for registered school nurses. My role as a school nurse in a busy children and families' team led me to consider the advantages and tensions of supporting pre-registration adult student nurses within our team. My reflections highlighted a number of key issues: these included the nature of school nursing work and particularly the large amount of safeguarding; capacity issues within a small team; and the relevance of the specialism to other nursing fields. My reflections took place prior to the introduction of the new standards of education for nursing (NMC, 2010). Of particular interest within the new standards is the focus on all nursing fields requiring exposure to community nursing. The standards also allow nurses to support and assess students from a different field of practice from their own. It will be interesting to see what effect the new standards have on mentoring pre-registration student nurses within the school nursing team.

The role of the school nurse has significantly altered over recent years. A series of deaths among vulnerable children in the United Kingdom has precipitated an increased focus on safeguarding activities for all professionals working with children. Following the tragic death of baby Peter Connolly in 2008 care applications for children rose by over 46 per cent in 2009 (Children and Family Court Advisory Service [CAFCAS], 2010). The CAFCAS described this as an 'unprecedented rise'. Safeguarding activities for the school nurse have also risen enormously. In a survey by the Royal College of Nursing (2009) 70 per cent of respondents working in state schools cited attending Child Protection Case Conferences as their most time-consuming activity, compared to 50 per cent in 2005. In addition, 29 per cent of respondents stated they would like to do less of this work and 54 per cent said they would like to increase their health promotion work. The extent of this mushrooming of safeguarding focus has yet to be fully recognised by policy makers and nurse education and will inevitably have an effect on the implementation of new pre-registration nursing curricula.

This focus within the school nurse caseload strongly influences their capacity to mentor and therefore assess pre-registration student nurses. This certainly isn't a problem for school nurses only. There are many examples in the current literature that highlight significant issues with capacity which impact on professionals' ability to undertake their day-to-day role, and this includes mentoring students. These issues were certainly reflected within the school nursing team in which I worked.

A review of the literature suggested that a possible solution to capacity issues could be found in utilising a team mentoring system. Gray and Smith (2000) found that students felt that it was not always necessary to work with their mentor. In fact, they found it positively useful to work with another nurse as they could see different styles of nursing at work, rather than just learning their mentor's approach to nursing. Hutchings et al. (2005: 953) concluded 'a two-mentor to one-learner support ratio is recommended to optimize mentor learner contact time'. Taylor (2008) identifies this system as already in place in her National Health Service Trust and

(Continued)

(Continued)

indeed this approach has been implemented in my own area. School nurses and Health Visitors will 'share' a student nurse according to the daily demands of their caseload. Currently this is an informal arrangement and can be potentially confusing for students The new NMC education standards (2010) will provide an opportunity to formalise this arrangement by embedding the structure within the curriculum. It can be argued that a mentor's caseload should be reduced prior to a student placement and subsequently should stay reduced for the duration of the placement. In view of the increased workload within my own team this was not implemented and school nurses managed their workload alongside supporting student nurses.

Hutchings et al. (2005) identify that the 'types of learners' allocated to a particular placement should be a key consideration. With this in mind, one way forward with mentoring in school nursing could be to think carefully about which students will benefit most from a school nursing placement. The NMC's (2008) 'due regard' principle says that mentors can only assess students on the same part of the register and the same field of practice as themselves. The new standards (NMC, 2010) now allow nurses to support students from all fields of practice apart from the final placement of the programme. This will undoubtedly lead to a more appropriate use of school nursing placements. There is a synergy between the role of the school nurse and that of the Mental Health Nurse, in that they both frequently work in the community and with families. In addition, the 'emotional labours' of these roles as explored by Smith (1992) have great similarities: there will now be an opportunity for other student nurses to benefit from school nursing placements and to link the generic skills shared with other fields. There are advantages as well to an adult pre-registration student having exposure to the school nurse role and to safeguarding considerations. Safeguarding is the province of all professionals with direct or indirect contact with children. However, spoke visits as opposed to hub placements may be a more appropriate use of the placement and the mentor, giving students a flavour of what is involved and an opportunity to practise generic skills without involving them in the 'emotional labour' of the role. Those nursing fields that would benefit from the increasing specialism of the role could then be mentored accordingly, with school nurse mentors providing appropriate levels of supervision and the assessment of more specialist skills.

The school nursing team in which I work is currently taking part in a root and branch evaluation of all practice placements in preparation for the introduction of the new NMC (2010) standards. This is an exciting opportunity to work alongside the higher education institution in structuring a placement circuit in which access to the generic skills shared by all nurses, including school nurses, can be balanced with the need to also expose some fields of nursing to a much more specialist set of skills and knowledge. The small steps taken thus far by the school nursing team (team mentoring, a review of capacity issues and consideration of the appropriateness of student placements) will assist this review. The new standards for pre-registration nurse education provide an excellent opportunity for practice staff and educationalists to explore a more imaginative utilisation of school nursing placements.

The learning organisation

It can be useful for mentors to consider the concept of the learning organisation when evaluating the effectiveness of their own environment. The concept of the learning organisation is most widely associated with the work of Donald Schön (1983) and more recently Peter Senge (1990). Schön was motivated by the ever-changing landscape of business to consider how organisations can survive in unstable times. For Schön (1983) one of the most important considerations was ensuring that businesses were able and ready to learn, that they could change quickly in response to economic, political and social change. This notion resembles the idea of continuing professional development and the assertion that one of the key skills required by health and social care students is the need to learn about learning. It is only by embracing this readiness to change that practitioners will continue to be effective. The work of Argyris and Schön (1978, 1996), particularly regarding feedback and single and double loop learning, is important as it suggests how organisations and practice can adapt and change. There have been a number of descriptions of a learning organisation. Rowden (2001), for example, has described four main characteristics of a learning organisation. These are a constant readiness to learn, continual planning, improvised implementation and action learning. The key feature of learning organisations is the flexibility and vision to change when change is needed. However, the concept of the learning organisation is not without its critics. In a sense the learning organisation can be viewed as an ideal, something to strive towards, and indeed there is very little empirical evidence supporting the learning organisation. The concept can be most useful for mentors when used to review the ways in which their own organisation reacts to change and how individuals and teams are supported through that process. In reviewing the characteristics of learning organisations in primary care, Rushmer et al. (2004) emphasise the significance of teams learning together and individuals sharing their learning for the benefit of the team. Students can be a dynamic ingredient in that structural learning and mentors in particular should be mindful of the mutuality of the learning that happens between them and mentees and utilise this for the benefit of the team.

The characteristics of an effective learning environment

What are the characteristics of an effective learning environment? At the start of this chapter it was suggested that the learning environment can be described as any place in which learning occurs. Although this is a good starting point when we wish to consider the management of the learning environment, and particularly maintaining quality within this aspect of the learning experience for students, this broad definition can also become less helpful. Can we describe an effective learning environment? It is clear from the discussion earlier that a good learning environment will share similar components. The quality of individual mentors is crucial to a successful student experience, so clearly one vital component of a good learning environment is good mentors who are skilled and enthusiastic in what they do. Mentors who are willing to structure learning for students, who can facilitate reflection in others, who are happy to be challenged about aspects of their own practice, and who will role model professional behaviour are essential to effective learning environments. There are, however, a number of other features that will also identify an effective environment for students and a number of studies have attempted to define the key characteristics of an effective learning environment. Research during the 1980s highlighted some interesting points regarding the learning environment, particularly work by Pembrey (1980), Orton (1981), Ogier (1982) and Fretwell (1983). These writers identified a number of characteristics that were regarded as important, and these can be summarised as:

- the use of a humanistic approach to learning;
- a good working team spirit in the clinical team;
- an efficient but flexible management style with teaching being recognised;
- teaching and learning support from qualified staff.

Although these studies were nursing focused and were conducted in a very different clinical setting from that which covers the current arrangements for student nurses they still give some useful indicators for effective learning environments. More recent work by Chan (2003) identified a number of significant factors in the Clinical Learning Environment Inventory:

- individualisation;
- innovation;
- involvement;
- personalisation;
- task orientation.

Chapter link

Check out how your practice area is audited. (See Chapter 5 for a further discussion on quality assurance mechanisms.)

These attempts at articulating what makes an effective environment for learning can be used by mentors to consider their own environment. In addition, as part of the quality processes of higher education institutions most pre-qualifying programmes will require placements to evaluate the effectiveness of the environment. In nursing and midwifery programmes this is a requirement of the Nursing and Midwifery Council (2008). In the north west of England a database has been created to manage placements and this also includes a placement audit. The electronic database is called the Placement Learning Support System (PLSS) and is used by universities in the north west to manage placements (www.plss.org.uk). The audit incorporated within the PLSS includes the following categories:

- diversity, values, beliefs and safety;
- improving and maintaining quality;
- resources, management and governance;
- teaching and learning;
- student/learner selection, progression and achievement;
- student and learner support;
- assessment;
- two categories pertaining specifically to Nursing and Midwifery Council standards.

This range of scales and audit tools demonstrates the necessity of getting the environment right. It is clear from the literature that there are key characteristics that should be attended to when evaluating the effectiveness of a learning environment. The range of audit tools also demonstrates the importance of quality processes within pre-qualifying programmes (an issue that is addressed in more detail in Chapter 5).

The case study below by Nicola Howard brings together some of these issues and highlights the factors that need to be considered when preparing a practice area for students. The use of an established audit tool, the need to invest in and value mentors and the need to prepare the physical environment for students are all considered here. Howard's study also emphasises the benefits to the practice setting of engaging fully with pre-registration student nurses.

CASE STUDY

Preparing a Community Mental Health Team for students – Nicola Howard

It is a rare opportunity nowadays for a service to actively participate in the structuring of a new endeavour in nurse education. The Community Mental Health Team (CMHT) in which I work had such an opportunity. Although the team had been involved in the ad hoc support of student nurses, the delivery of a pre-registration mental health nurse programme had ceased over twenty years ago. The team did also have significant experience of supporting other health and social care students, particularly social work students. In September 2009 we accepted our first degree-level pre-registration mental health nursing students. The first steps in approaching this required a robust scrutiny of the learning environment. There also needed to be a re-establishment of the link between academic staff and practice staff. In order to approach this issue an educational audit was completed. A team was assembled to approach all of the prospective placements to address issues such as numbers of mentors for students, how many students could be accommodated, the learning opportunities within placements, and the education profile of staff and their preparedness for supporting students. The Practice Placement Support System (PLSS) audit tool was completed and the relevant data compiled. This audit gave a full picture of the readiness of placements and practice staff and highlighted the preparation that would be needed prior to placements commencing.

The issues identified in the CMHT were similar to other areas and covered staff education issues, appropriate learning opportunities within the team and the appropriateness of physical resources. Training needs were critically reviewed, especially mentor status. This highlighted a good number of qualified mentors; however, they all required updates to ensure they were aware of the new mentor standards and changes in nurse education. This also highlighted where further training would be beneficial. It had been some time since the mental health service had been used in pre-registration education and there had been many changes in the interim; probably the most fundamental of these was the move from local schools of nursing to the university setting. Locally we made the decision to move to all-degree education earlier than the United Kingdom so all of our mental health students would be undergraduates. To assist with this transition a member of the team was appointed as a Practice Guide (for more information on this role see Pauline Keenan's case study in Chapter 3). The majority of practitioners embraced the higher academic level and took personal advantage of courses offered at academic levels 6 and 7.

The emphasis within the current nursing curriculum on concepts such as critical reflection, inter-professional learning (IPL) and the notion of students as adult learners who are actively encouraged to question, reflect upon and challenge practice was new to many mentors. It was imperative that the CMHT was aware of these changes and able to provide learning opportunities in order to ensure students were able to meet these requirements. The CMHT provided an excellent opportunity for examples of inter-professional learning and the educational audit was able to highlight this feature of our work. This is crucial as practice placements are critical to the experiences of student nurses and must reflect the provision of health care needs and the requirements of professional registration. These requirements are reflected in even more detail in the new pre-registration nursing standards for competence and standards for education (NMC, 2010).

The physical resources within a placement area also play a vital role in ensuring an effective learning environment. The CMHT were keen to ensure that students felt welcomed and included within the team from the beginning of a placement. Arrangements were therefore made to ensure the environment was ready for students. Educational resources were prepared, desk space and a computer were made available, and a student welcome pack was devised. This pack consisted of a 'who's who' list with relevant contact details and a description of various departments, plus a diary or diary sheets, note pad and pen. These arrangements ensured that students felt they were part of the team from early in their placement.

Prior to attending a practice placement students will have spent time in an academic setting and their practice placement should allow them the

(Continued)

(Continued)

chance to link theory with practice. A mentor therefore needs to be familiar with a student's programme of study and also their experience prior to the placements. Practitioners In the CMHT have come to realise that by ensuring the environment is appropriate they can play a significant part in the development of student mental health nurses.

The experience of preparing the CMHT for pre-registration students has highlighted the many benefits of having students in the community team. Foremost among these is the involvement of team members in mentorship updates and nurse education generally. This has encouraged a number of practitioners to review their own education needs; this has undoubtedly increased their confidence and made them better able to relate theory to practice. Students are encouraged to challenge and question and thus it is necessary to be aware of current research, government reports and innovative techniques so that these can be explained confidently to students. Professionals in the placement area are role models for learners and as a result need to be conscious of their own actions, behaviours and attitudes. The need for self-awareness and the ability to participate in reflection are an advantage as these are skills that students also require. The re-introduction of the pre-registration mental health nursing programme has enabled mentors and placements to contribute to the future of mental health nursing locally. The development of the learning environment has been an evolving learning experience and one from which nurse students, mentors, professionals and the practice placement have benefited.

Howard's case study really does unpick what needs to be considered when constructing an environment for learning. Simple things like creating space for students, assembling a welcome pack and providing well prepared mentors are key contributions towards a good learning experience. Furthermore, this case study emphasises the necessity of mentors being up to date both on mentorship issues and their own practice. As in Dunajewski's case study this emphasis on education and further professional development can positively influence the entire team.

Chapter summary

Evaluating the learning environment is a crucial element of mentorship as the quality of the learning experience is inextricably linked to that environment. This chapter has defined what is meant by 'the learning environment' and has suggested that health and social care pre-qualifying programmes should utilise a diverse range of placement opportunities. These placement opportunities are embedded in the notion of learning from experience. Regardless of where that learning takes places there are key elements for mentors to consider when managing the learning environment. These include the nature of the mentor–mentee relationship and the potential impact of the environment upon that relationship, the requirement to incorporate opportunities for reflection within practice learning and the need to evaluate the learning environment against established criteria.

The complexities of deconstructing the nature of the learning environment can be seen in the need to refer the reader to a number of other chapters in the book. The learning environment cannot be understood in isolation from key concepts such as relationships, reflection, experiential learning and evaluation. The learning environment is a key factor in supporting students in the practice setting and mentors should embrace the complexities of managing the environment to ensure a rich learning experience is cultivated.

Reflective activity

Having read the chapter you should be more able to consider your own environment and evaluate the effectiveness of that environment for learning. Take a look at the box below and use the headings to reflect on the environment in which you mentor:

- How can managers/leaders demonstrate their commitment to learning?
- Are learners orientated to the team/environment on commencement of their placement?
- Are you able to designate time to facilitate learner reflection? How do you ensure this?
- What specific learning opportunities are available in your practice area?
- What audit processes does your practice area participate in?
- What learning resources are available to learners in your team?
- How do learners formally evaluate your practice area?

References

Argyris, C. and Schön, D. (1978) *Organisational Learning I: A Theory of Action Perspective.* Reading, MA: Addison Weslcy.

Argyris, C. and Schön, D. (1996) *Organisational Learning II: Theory, Method and Practice.* Reading, MA: Addison Wesley.

Baillee, L. (1999) 'Preparing adult branch students for their management role as staff nurses: an action research project', *Journal of Nursing Management,* 7: 225–234.

Benner, P. (1984) *From Novice to Expert.* Reading, MA: Addison Wesley.

Chan, D. (2003) 'Validation of the clinical learning environment inventory', *Western Journal of Nursing Research,* 25: 519–532.

Children and Family Court Advisory Services (CAFCAS) (2010) *Care Demand Statistics.* Available at www.cafcass.gov.uk/PDF/0910%20Q1%20care%20demand%20update%202009%2007%2016.pdf (last accessed 15 April 2010).

Clarke, D.J. and Copeland, L. (2003) 'Developing working practice through work-based learning', *Nurse Education in Practice,* 3 (4): 236–244.

Dewey, J. (1938) *Experience and Education.* New York: Collier.

Duffy, K. (2003) *Failing Students: A Qualitative Study of Factors that Influence the Decisions Regarding Assessment of Students' Competence in Practice.* Glasgow: Caledonian University and Nursing and Midwifery Council.

Eraut, M. (2004) 'Informal learning in the workplace', *Studies in Continuing Education,* 26 (2): 247–273.

Fretwell, J.E. (1983) *Ward Teaching and Learning.* London: RCN.

Graham, I.W. (1995) 'Reflective practice: using the action learning group mechanism', *Nurse Education Today,* 15: 28–32.

Gray, M.A. and Smith, L.N. (2000) 'The qualities of an effective mentor from the student nurse's perspective: findings from a longitudinal qualitative study', *Journal of Advanced Nursing,* 32 (6): 1542–1549.

Henderson, A., Twentyman, M., Eaton, E., Creedy, D., Stapleton, P. and Lloyd, B. (2009) 'Creating supportive clinical learning environments: an intervention study', *Journal of Clinical Nursing,* 19: 177–182.

Hutchings, A., Williams, G. and Humphreys, A. (2005) 'Supporting learners in clinical practice: capacity issues', *Journal of Clinical Nursing,* 14: 945–955.

Kolb, D.A. (1984) *Experiential Learning.* Englewood Cliffs, NJ: Prentice- Hall.

McIntosh, A. (2011) 'Evaluation'. In A. McIntosh, J. Gidman and E. Mason-Whitehead (eds), *Key Concepts in Healthcare Education.* London: Sage.

Mezirow, J. (2000) *Learning as Transformation: Critical Perspectives on a Theory in Progress.* San Francisco, CA: Jossey-Bass.

Nursing and Midwifery Council (2008) *Standards to Support Learning and Assessment in Practice* (2nd edn). London: NMC.

Nursing and Midwifery Council (2010) *Standards for Pre-Registration Nursing Education.* Available at http://standards.nmc-uk.org/PreReg Nursing/statutory/background/Pages/Introduction.aspx (last accessed 27 March 2011).

O'Connor, A. (2001) *Clinical Instruction and Evaluation: A Teaching Resource* (2nd edn). Sudbury, MA: Jones & Bartlett.

Ogier, M.E. (1982) *An Ideal Sister?* London: RCN.

Orton, H.D. (1981) *Ward Learning Climate: A Study of the Role of the Ward Sister in Relation to Student Nurse Learning on the Ward.* London: RCN.

Pembrey, S.E.M. (1980) *The Ward Sister – Key to Nursing.* London: RCN.

Price, B. (2003) 'Building a rapport with the learner', *Nursing Standard,* 19 (22): 1–2.

Rowden, R.W. (2001) 'The learning organisation and strategic change', *Advanced Management Journal,* 66 (3): 11–24.

Royal College of Nursing (2009) *RCN: School Nurses Feeling the Strain of Public Health Demands.* Available at www.rcn.org.uk/newsevents/ news/article/uk/rcn_school_nurses_feeling_the_strain_of_public_health_ demands (last accessed 30 April 2010).

Rushmer, R., Lough, M., Wilkinson, J. and Davies, H.T.O. (2004) 'Introducing the learning practice – I: the characteristics of learning organisations in primary care', *Journal of Evaluation in Clinical Practice,* 10 (3): 375–386.

Schön, D.A. (1983) *Beyond the Stable State: Public and Private Learning in a Changing Society.* Harmondsworth: Penguin.

Senge, P.M. (1990) *The Fifth Discipline: The Art and Practice of the Learning Organization.* London: Random House.

Smith, P. (1992) *The Emotional Labour of Nursing.* London: Macmillan.

Taylor, J. (2008) 'Are you a good mentor?', *Nursing times.net.* Available at www. nursingtimes.net/are-you-a-good-mentor/1795628.article (last accessed 19 May 2010).

7 The Context of Practice

Case studies: Samanthia Harley, Angela Anderson, Finbarr Murphy and Audrey Craig

We have established in previous chapters that a mentor's skills, qualities and characteristics are essential prerequisites to a good placement. However, in Chapter 6 we discussed the environment's importance in terms of student learning. One of the key considerations when determining the quality of the learning environment is the extent to which the professionals who work within that environment are engaged in contemporary practice. In addition to this mentors and educationalists also need to be cognisant of the political and professional pressures that will inevitably have an impact on professional practice. The last decade has seen an incredible amount of change both in health and social care organisation and practice and the social context in which professionals act. An increasingly litigious society has arguably fostered a defensive attitude in many practitioners and increasing financial pressures on a global scale are having an impact on health and social care provision. The first two case studies in this chapter demonstrate in different ways the changing nature of health and social care. In the first of these Samanthia Harley discusses the impact of unregistered practitioners on midwifery care and the potential tensions and challenges of supporting learning with this group of staff. In the second Angela Anderson gives a description of her career pathway and the ways in which changing expectations have impacted on career progression in nursing. Later in the chapter Finbarr Murphy, a social worker in a drug and alcohol team, uses his case study to show the political nature of health and social care activity and the significance of this for students. This becomes particularly important when students may have previously held taken-for-granted assumptions about the client group concerned. The final case study by Audrey Craig, also a social worker, shows how time spent incorporating the principles of group supervision within a morning team meeting can benefit individuals, the organisation, and ultimately the service user.

The chapter will consider the impact of the context of practice on two levels. Firstly, we will evaluate some key changes in professional practice and the impact these changes have on practice education, and in particular review the changing face of contemporary health and social care and discuss what this means for current learners and their mentors. Secondly, we will examine the impact of these changes on mentors and what it means for them to manage practice learning amid continual change. A notable feature of contemporary professional practice is the ability to manage change and indeed lead change, and this is an increasing focus within the education outcomes of professional programmes. Mentors will be expected to play a crucial role within this change. Two aspects of professional practice that learners will be exposed to is the increase in inter-professional working and the rise in importance of service user involvement in both practice and professional education programmes. The chapter will evaluate the impact of both of these aspects of care and the ways in which mentors can ensure that student learning is structured to incorporate both. The chapter will begin with a reminder about the importance of high quality practice placements within professional education programmes.

Chapter learning objectives

By the end of the chapter the reader should be able to:

- critically evaluate the nature and importance of practice learning;
- critically analyse the impact of key social and political changes on health and social care practice;
- critically reflect upon the importance of inter-professional and service user involvement within a health and social care context.

The importance and complexities of practice

In the introduction to this book we mentioned the pressures on mentors to not only speak about what it is they do (to know it) but also to demonstrate the skills that make up their craft (to do it). As it stands this is a complex undertaking, but when we then take into consideration the chaos that can exist in a practice setting, the mentors' management of this complexity becomes even more remarkable. Yet the importance of getting this right cannot be underestimated as practice accounts for up to half of most professional pre-qualifying programmes. The Health and Care Professions Council (2012) emphasise the necessity of having quality practice placements and the need for strong partnership working. In Chapter 6 we highlighted the features of an effective learning environment and demonstrated the learning environment's impact on student learning. The context of that practice environment has never been more fluid, thus making mentorship a continually evolving activity. There are many accounts in the literature of barriers to good mentoring. Gainsbury's (2010) study highlights that a shortage of staff, a lack of time and increasing work pressures all play a part in poor mentoring, particularly where mentors were failing to fail student nurses.

Chapter link

Review the description of an effective learning environment in Chapter 6. In what ways might the context of practice affect the environment?

Our first case study examines the complexities and challenges associated with supporting reluctant learners. Very often we will make assumptions that adult learners are ready and motivated to learn and yet this is not always the case. Harley discusses the importance of understanding what the barriers may be to students engaging in learning by looking at the difficulties encountered when supporting a midwifery care assistant. The introduction of midwifery care assistants is relatively recent and highlights the differing responses to contemporary health and social care practice.

Supporting the reluctant learner – Samanthia Harley

The role of the modern midwife, along with many other health and social care roles, has changed and adapted to reflect the evolving needs and expectations of service users. These developments have impacted directly on the delivery of midwifery care. Specific issues, including the recruitment and retention of qualified midwives, the requirements for greater inter-professional working, ever-increasing technical advances, and the implementation of evidence-based practice, are challenging modern service delivery. One of the responses to these challenges within midwifery services has been the introduction of the midwifery care assistant. The midwifery care assistant is an unregistered carer who supports the midwife and invariably will undertake extra training in specific clinical procedures.

I am a midwife working in a busy midwifery department. Although we support a number of learners within the environment facilitating the learning of the midwifery care assistant has at times been a particular challenge. This case study will discuss the challenges associated with the reluctant learner, what may be the causes of an individual's reluctance to engage in learning and possible strategies that mentors could employ in order to engage reluctant learners.

The continuing development of midwifery care assistants can be viewed as an excellent opportunity for the individual concerned to extend their knowledge and improve the care they deliver. Knowles et al. (2005) describe the characteristics of adult learners and suggest that adults are particularly motivated to learn when that learning is relevant to what they do. Smith and Sadler-Smith (2006) also suggest that some adults will be fearful of engaging in academic processes. Certainly I have had experience of midwifery care assistants who are fearful of commencing further studies connected to their work and this can sometimes be perceived as reluctance. Some have described their negative experiences during school years and the negative impact of those experiences on their current attitude to learning. There is a danger here that a mentor may not find out this information, particularly if there isn't sufficient time to mentor or time has not been invested in building an effective relationship. It has now become an expectation that midwifery care assistants will be involved in more clinical activities and so need to be prepared to do this (Department of Health [DH], 2000, 2006). This can potentially cause conflict and mentors need to recognise this and manage it effectively.

(Continued)

(Continued)

Knowles et al. (2005) stated that a readiness to learn may be stimulated by helping individuals to identify their current needs and aspirations and what was needed to achieve those aspirations. This is a skilled job for mentors and one which requires them to invest time. This will inevitably help the mentoring relationship and hopefully ensure some of the educational barriers are broken down. A mentor should endeavour to use praise at every opportunity, and particularly with fearful learners, as self-esteem can be increased and in this way the engagement can continue. Emphasising any extrinsic factors that may motivate the learner can also prove useful, for instance any pay incentives that may be connected to the learning being undertaken.

Helping another person to learn can be a great privilege and one of the most rewarding aspects of a midwife mentor's job. However, a learner that is reluctant to engage in the learning process can be a particular challenge for mentors. To ensure that the mentoring relationship will be both effective and rewarding, mentors need to invest time in uncovering any issues that may affect a mentee's motivation to learn.

The narrative for recent health and social care provision has undoubtedly been one characterised by change. From the publication of the NHS Plan (DH, 2000) and the range of national service frameworks, to the impact of high profile safeguarding cases, health and social care professionals have needed to adjust in response to changing political and professional drivers. These drivers have culminated in services that seem to be in a constant state of flux. Changes have also occurred in the ways in which health and social care professionals work and in new career pathways. These changes then impact not only on how students understand their role as members of a new profession but also on the ways in which mentors will work. It is vital that mentors help students to translate these changes and make sense of them within the learning context. The shift in health care from the acute setting to the community setting is a particular challenge in pre-registration nurse education. The need to incorporate a greater emphasis on public health within the pre-registration nursing curriculum and more public health practice experience is high on the professional agenda. In our next case study Angela Anderson discusses her varied roles in nursing and the similarity that exists between the skills related to effective mentorship and those identified as essential community nursing skills.

Using mentorship skills to aid transition into a community team – Angela Anderson

My role as a registered adult nurse has allowed me to enjoy a number of varied roles both in an acute setting (medical and surgical wards) and within a community children and families' team working in the health visiting team, as well as more recently as part of the school nursing team. The knowledge, skills and values I practised as a mentor in the acute setting have transferred very easily into the community team. What was less easy for me was to recognise my role as a health promoter within that setting. However, when I compared the two sets of skills as a mentor and health promoter I started to recognise some distinct similarities between these. This short case study will share my reflections on the shared knowledge and skills base of the two roles.

The Prime Minister's Commission Report (2010) on the future of nursing and midwifery and work by the World Health Organization [WHO] (1998) identified health promotion and education as key roles for nurses. Indeed, Florence Nightingale wrote that nurses should act as educators in order to promote health. My experience of working in busy acute areas has been that health promotion is not prioritised within busy inpatient practice areas where very often a shortage of staff and complex health needs are evident. However, Scriven and Garman (2005) argue that nurses have the knowledge base and the personal contact with patients to enable them to engage in health promotional activities. The ultimate goal of health promotion is to enable patients to make informed choices about lifestyle issues and health interventions. It seemed to me that this idea of educating and empowering was very similar to the activities I did as a mentor. This realisation enabled me to feel more confident about my role as a health promoter in a community setting. A mentor's key skill lies in establishing effective relationships with students and empowering them to make appropriate choices. This is also essential to health promotion activity. Assessment and appropriate feedback skills are also key in both roles.

As nursing careers inevitably change to fit with reconfigured services nurses need to identify generic skills that cut across service boundaries. I found as I moved from an acute hospital setting to a community setting that the skills I had developed as a mentor were invaluable. I not only used these skills to support learners within the community team I was also able to transfer these skills to service specific aspects of my role as a community practitioner.

The story of recent health and social care provision, as Harley and Anderson demonstrate in their case studies, is undoubtedly one that is characterised by change. This change adds to the challenges faced by mentors who are striving to facilitate learning in practice settings. Waters (2001) argues there are three crucial aspects within practice learning: it is the place where professional skills, knowledge and values are acquired; it is the place where practice is theorised and theory is practised; and it is where learners go through a process of encul-turisation (namely, they learn how to be professional). A complexity within practice learning is the nature of learning 'on the shopfloor'. Very often students will be anxious about getting it wrong in practice and so they will require support to enable them to relax within the team. Likewise mentors must structure student learning and specifically do so in order to ensure that programme learning outcomes are met. Practice, however, can often be unpredictable and mentors need to be sufficiently vigilant to spot opportunistic learning. This type of learning can have real meaning for students, especially when the experience is consolidated with time for reflection. In Chapter 3 Anna Turco gives some simple but effective tips on how mentors can structure time for reflection within their busy day. The importance of social learning theory becomes apparent when we consider the nature of learning in practice. The principles of this theory rely on the observer being able to take on board the actions of another and crucially the observed (the mentor) being able to model best practice. In contrast to pure behaviourist theory, social learning theory suggests that individuals have the potential to influence their own behaviour. The implications of this for mentors are noteworthy. We have identified that modelling appropriate skills, knowledge and values is an essential skill within mentoring. However, social learning theory emphasises the real significance of this skill. Mentors are able to construct situations in which learners can observe practice situations and learn best practice. This is particularly worthwhile in relation to modelling professional behaviours. When linked with time to reflect on what has been observed this becomes a really powerful way of learning. In addition though it highlights the pressures on mentors when supporting learners and the need to be conscious of their behaviour and the messages that are shared, both explicitly and implicitly, about professional practice.

Chapter link

Take some time to review the concepts of social learning theory. (Take a look at Chapter 3 for a full discussion.)

One of the differences with learning in the practice setting rather than a classroom setting is the public nature of that learning. In many ways classrooms can provide a safe haven for educationalists (although it may not always feel like it!). Learning in a practice setting happens in front of service users, colleagues, carers and other health and social care professionals. Very often there will be an audience for that learning. This will inevitably have an influence on both mentors and learners. A mentor will be exposing their professional knowledge and behaviours to the scrutiny of others. A learner can also feel the pressure of needing to 'get it right' not only for the mentor but also for whoever else is listening. Mentors should be mindful of these factors and consider the environment in which questions are asked. Perhaps for less experienced learners this exposure should be minimal. More experienced learners need to be confident in dealing with this public scrutiny as it is very often the nature of professional practice once qualified, therefore increasing learners' exposure to this type of scrutiny should be a gradual process.

One further complexity to teaching in the practice setting is the notion of risk and risk management. This can cause some anxiety for mentors and indeed they can potentially jeopardise the learning that is made available to mentees by curtailing their experience. Clark and Cox (2011) highlight how delegation is valuable within the context of professional accountability. As professionals we are ultimately accountable for the appropriateness of the aspects of care we delegate to learners. There are a number of key aspects associated with delegating to learners. First and foremost mentors must be confident that each learner is competent enough to complete that delegated activity. This means that thorough initial assessments are paramount at the commencement of a practice placement. In Chapter 4 we discuss the importance of initial assessments for the appropriate structuring of learning activities; however, this assessment should also be the basis for decisions concerning the delegation of activities. Mentors should be certain that a learner is competent to undertake activities safely, that they fully understand what is being delegated and that they are aware that they should verbalise any concerns they may have regarding that care activity. Mentors should also be prepared to check that the delegated activities have been completed to a satisfactory standard. Stuart (2007) suggests that nurse mentors are professionally accountable for the following aspects of mentorship:

- their own standards of professional practice;
- the standards of care delivered by student nurses;
- what is taught, learned and assessed;

- their own standards of teaching and assessment;
- the judgements they make about student performance.

Mentors must be aware of their accountability and responsibilities when supporting learning and must also be able to manage any potential risks in a proactive manner.

Interprofessional learning and working

The nature of health and social care practice is changing. One of the most significant changes is the extent to which different professional groups are expected to work together. This expectation has had an impact on professional qualifying programmes. There is an increasing emphasis on exposing learners to the complexities of inter-professional working, both within the practice setting and within the academic setting.

Interprofessional learning (IPL) is defined by Hammick et al. (2007: 7) 'as learning arising from interaction between members (or students) of two or more professions. This may be a product of interprofessional education or happen spontaneously in the workplace or in education settings'. The United Kingdom Centre for the Advancement of Interprofessional Education simply defines it as 'the occasions when two or more professions learn from and about each other to improve collaboration and the quality of care' (Walsh et al., 2005: 231).

The concept of IPL has had a long history although we tend to associate it with contemporary health and social care practice. IPL is an excellent example of the impact of political, professional and social drivers on health and social care practice. Barr and Sharland (2012) argue that interprofessional education has been a key element of the political agenda for over a decade, while Worsley (2011) documents the large numbers of enquiries and policy directives that have impacted on IPL.

It is important that we distinguish between two specific aspects of IPL. Firstly, there is the notion, evidenced in a number of government-driven initiatives, that IPL will encourage professions to learn and understand the common ground that exists between them. This is based on an assumption that those who are working in health and social care share a set of generic skills and knowledge and so 'common learning' is the purpose. The second notion of IPL is that there are enormous benefits to the various health and social care professions learning with, from and about each other. Barr et al. (2012) suggest that the 'common learning' approach, particularly when it tries to enforce a 'generic health culture', is problematic. A review of qualifying programmes in social work and nursing illustrates some of the tensions within IPL. The Nursing and Midwifery Council (2010) in their new standards for pre-registration nurse education have emphasised the requirements for both intraprofessional learning (between fields of nursing) and interprofessional learning alongside students from other professional programmes. Indeed the NMC have also relaxed the 'due regard' requirement for nursing mentors, thus allowing those from other professions (after appropriate preparation) to support nursing students. The introduction of the social work degree in 2003 included collaborative working and learning with others as a key aspect of the programme. Interestingly, more recently The College of Social Work in their standards for practice educators (2012) have stipulated that by 2015 all social work students must be supported by practice educators who are also registered social workers, thus establishing due regard within social work education.

Yet despite recognition of its value there are real obstacles to establishing effective IPL. Barr et al. (2012) have put forward three key challenges that they feel need to be addressed. They suggest that:

- there needs to be an agreement amongst professional bodies regarding the initial requirements of students in order to create an interprofessional curriculum;
- educators need to ensure that this agreement works in the long term and not just the short term;
- evidence-based implementation strategies are required to ensure the effectiveness of these programmes.

Chapter link

See Chapter 4 for a further discussion of the implications of interprofessional mentorship to assessment and due regard.

The IPL debate is important for practice mentors as they are required to integrate what has been taught in the classroom regarding IPL with what is seen in practice. In many ways the nature of contemporary service delivery means that learners will inevitably work alongside other professionals. It is crucial for mentors to bring to the fore the challenges and benefits of this.

A further aspect of interprofessional learning is interprofessional mentorship. As we have discussed throughout this book, supervising students in a practice setting is a crucial aspect of every professional's role. In this way health and social care professionals will have already gained good insight into the role of mentor. However, there can be anxieties when mentors are asked to support students coming from professions that are different from their own. Marshall and Gordon describe interprofessional mentorship as 'occasions when a health and social professional facilitates interprofessional learning and supervises and assesses students in the practice setting' (2005: 39). Mentors' skills when assessing students from other professions will be identical to those required to support students from their own profession. The skills for effective relationship building, including excellent interpersonal skills and the ability to motivate and be confident about their own skills and knowledge, are key to both types of mentorship. Clearly, though, one activity that will be different when mentoring students from other professions is the emphasis on a specific professional knowledge base and values framework. The benefits of interprofessional mentoring will come about as a result of students learning with, from and about other professions. Marshall et al. (2005) argue that shared learning outcomes across professions would be a useful addition to professional education programmes rather than relying on profession specific outcomes alone. Marshall et al. (2005: 41) go on to summarise the key messages for interprofessional mentorship:

- interprofessional mentorship is a vehicle for developing integrated, modernised services;
- the key skills required are transferable from current practice;
- interprofessional mentorship already exists in an informal format;
- patients and service users must be placed at the centre of interprofessional learning experiences;
- common learning outcomes provide a focus for interprofessional mentorship;
- interprofessional mentorship enhances but does not replace uni-professional mentorship.

In the next case study Finbarr Murphy describes his attempts to integrate learning for social work students within an inter-professional drug and alcohol team. Murphy demonstrates both the complexities of this environment and the tremendous opportunities available to learners within this particular practice setting. The beginning of the study also highlights the political nature of health and social care, namely that professionals do not act in a value-free context. Drug and alcohol services are a good example of a service which will inevitably challenge the taken-for-granted assumptions of learners. As Murphy demonstrates, this therefore inevitably offers lots of opportunities for mentors and learners to undertake reflection, in particular within the affective domain.

The nature of inter-professional working in a drug and alcohol team – Finbarr Murphy

CASE STUDY

My role as a social worker in a multi-professional drug and alcohol team has provided many opportunities to support social work students. This type of team affords numerous occasions for social work students to enhance their knowledge, skills and professional values. However, this type of practice placement is not without its challenges. Drug and alcohol use and misuse will have varying impacts upon individuals, families and society, and these issues feature regularly in the news media. Indeed substance 'harms' have been well documented (Nutt et al., 2010). Political responses to these issues have been somewhat ambivalent, given that in 2008 in the United Kingdom there were 1,952 drug-related deaths (St George's University of London, 2009) and 9,031 alcohol-related deaths (BBC, 2010). The stringency of the legislation regarding drug misuse is in marked contrast to that for alcohol misuse; however, the alcohol industry provides governments and political parties with significant revenue. It is arguable that the dismissal of Professor Nutt from the Advisory Council on the Misuse of Drugs in 2010 provides evidence of political reactions to public opinion rather than actions based on scientific evidence of drug 'harms'. Nevertheless, politicians have endorsed strategies to address drug- and alcohol-related crime and disorder, and the need for treatment and support interventions.

The General Social Care Council (GSCC) (2005) supports the development of knowledge and skills for social workers who need to respond to drug and alcohol problems. A brief review of current mainstream social work texts highlights the importance of upholding professional values when working with disadvantaged groups such as older people. However, these texts do not directly address the ethical dilemmas and value conflicts which occur in working with people who have alcohol and/or drug problems.

(Continued)

(Continued)

For example, how might a social worker respond to an older person who is chemically dependent on prescribed drugs? Galvani and Forrester note that social workers are likely to have caseloads almost half of which will be clients with drug and/or alcohol problems, and these authors contend 'that social work courses tend to provide so little training on this issue, is inexcusable ... they are not being properly trained for their profession' (2008: 30).

Given this social and political context, a social work placement with a multi-professional drug and alcohol team presents mentors and students with significant challenges, particularly when addressing the gap between student knowledge and required professional standards. A drug and alcohol team will often comprise medical, nursing, psychology, occupational therapy, probation, social work, administrative and managerial disciplines. Social work knowledge occupies a continuum between the practical task-centred approach and humanistic psychological approaches. Howard et al. (2007: 561) suggest that 'it is not readily apparent that pedagogical practices in social work have changed significantly in recent years'.

The drug and alcohol team provides mentors and social work students with an opportunity to transcend the boundaries between pedagogy and andragogy. Given the time constraints of student placements, I am aware that it is necessary to implement a range of teaching and learning strategies to enable students to develop a body of knowledge or a set of skills that will fulfil the expected learning outcomes. During the initial phase of the placement I will very often use a pedagogical approach which may incorporate specific teaching strategies. These teaching strategies are aimed at producing cognitive, affective and psychomotor outcomes. Each student will be welcomed into the team and offered an introduction which includes: information-giving about the service philosophy, codes of conduct and the team personnel; client profiling; service delivery and eligibility criteria; departmental policies and procedures; information systems; and community resources. A practice portfolio will record a student's knowledge, skills, observed practice and evaluation. At this point the aim is for students to get a sense of the team and the differing contributions made by professionals within that team.

The cognitive domain may be addressed through mentor and student reflection on observations of other professionals' responses to alcohol and drug use. Students will be required to gather information in relation to good practice and access training DVDs, internet resources and textbooks in relation to drug and alcohol issues. Thereafter an andragogical approach may be incorporated in order to assist student reflection on these practice experiences, and address students' caseload experiences.

The affective domain includes the values and attitudes within the learning environment and the sometimes contrasting personal attitudes and beliefs of students. I have used the Social Work and Substance Use Questionnaire (Galvani et al., 2008) within my own placement area. Utilising this questionnaire along with taking time to discuss and reflect on the results can be effective when addressing those aspects of students' perceptions which have been influenced by news media coverage rather than evidence. For example, one student had reservations about assisting a client to make benefit claims, assuming that the additional monies would be used to fund further drug misuse. This student was helped through discussion and reflection to appreciate that clients have welfare benefit entitlements regardless of how they choose to use those benefits. This was a very good example of how personal and professional assumptions and values can contribute to further oppression and disadvantage. This learning is also difficult to achieve in a classroom.

The psychomotor domain involves activity and/or the use of motor skills, for example learning how to undertake a drug screening. Such learning may require students to engage in imitation, follow a sequence of instructions accurately and consistently, and ultimately, to perform such actions automatically. Students will be allocated a small caseload, under supervision, and as a result mentoring can assist in promoting learning in terms of knowledge, skills or attitudinal change. In this way mentoring enables students to relate abstract theory with concrete experience.

In summary, a practice placement within a multi-professional environment presents a range of challenges. For social work students learning must occur across a multitude of dimensions. In terms of their personal, professional and social development, students must reflect upon their own values and skills, challenge their assumptions, and document their learning and change. They also need to develop effective working relationships with a vulnerable client group, something which requires them to challenge personal values that are often influenced by media and/or political perspectives. Similarly, there are challenges for mentors as they attempt to enable learning and development within a multi-professional environment, promote an appreciation of professional diversity and maintain effective partnerships with colleagues from other disciplines, challenge practices, and coordinate multi-professional resources for the benefit of both students and clients. It is these unique challenges that also provide rich opportunities for learning.

Murphy's case study highlights a number of interesting points for mentors. He articulates the political nature of social work and the ways in which mentors can harness these tensions to enhance student learning. In particular, he has emphasised how these situations can help learners to evaluate and re-evaluate their taken-for-granted assumptions about practice. A potential benefit of learning in an inter-professional team is the notion that inter-professional mentorship will occur and thus broaden students' exposure to the articulation of professional values in practice. The case study shows that by thinking about learning in terms of the three domains (cognitive, affective and psychomotor) mentors can effectively facilitate structured learning experiences amid potentially chaotic practice environments.

Service user and carer involvement in learning

The involvement of service users and carers within professional education programmes has become a significant driver over recent years. It is generally agreed that increased collaborative working with service users and carers will benefit learners and ultimately have a positive effect on service delivery. However, there is much debate regarding the most effective ways of achieving this. As we discussed with IPL earlier in the chapter, universities are now required to involve service users and carers in the planning, design, delivery and evaluation of their programmes. The extent to which this happens differs from institution to institution and programme to programme. The complexities of involving service users and carers within the academic component of a programme are well documented and to some extent these are lessened for practice mentors. Practice is the place where learners will interact with service users and carers on a daily basis. However, for practice mentors it is important to understand the emphasis on this involvement and to consider ways in which service users and carers can play a meaningful role in all aspects of learners' practice experience. In Chapter 4 we consider the ways in which service users and carers can inform the assessment process in practice and this continues to be a complex aspect of service user and carer involvement.

Chapter link

Consider the benefits and challenges of including service users and carers in the assessment process. (Have a look at Chapter 4 for a further discussion.)

The Commission for Social Care Inspection (CSCI) (2007) has produced eight principles that universities should consider when involving service users and carers. These principles can be summarised as follows:

- be clear about the purpose of involving service users and carers;
- agree with service users and carers the ways in which they will be involved;
- service users and carers should choose how they wish to become involved;
- give appropriate feedback about the outcome of their involvement;
- recognise and overcome barriers to implementation;
- make efforts to include the widest range of people;
- value the contribution, expertise and time of service users and carers;
- use the lessons learnt from service user and carer involvement to influence change.

The concept of involving service users and carers in professional education programmes has had a long history. The notion of individualised, collaborative care based on choice is a key feature of contemporary health and social care practice, although over the last decade or so government policy and professional interest has embraced this concept more fully, making it a key feature on the professional and political agenda. McIntosh et al. (2011) discuss in some detail the key policy documents extolling the benefits of service user and carer involvement. Sawyer (2005) also argues that mutual trust is the key characteristic of partnership working and to achieve this there needs to be open communication, shared values and goals, shared risk, joint problem solving and a no-blame culture.

The work of Tew et al. (2004) identifies a list of potential areas in which service users and carers can be involved in education and training, and while this report is specifically for mental health education and training it can be applied to other health and social care professions. Tew et al. argue that there is a spectrum of service user and carer involvement which includes:

- the direct delivery of learning and teaching;
- course/module planning;
- the recruitment and selection of students;
- practice learning;
- student assessment;
- course evaluation;
- service users and carers on courses as participants.

They go on to emphasise that good preparation and support are key aspects to service user and carer involvement and also discuss the importance of shared partnership values. A number of strategies can be employed by mentors to ensure the full involvement of service users and carers. Ensuring their own practice places service users and carers at the centre of care resulting in the role modelling of collaborative partnership working which is essential. Mentors should also be mindful of ensuring that learners are encouraged to reflect on this aspect of care and to consider their own values in relation to care giving. McIntosh et al. (2011) suggest the involvement of service users and carers can be a troublesome activity as it highlights crucial issues arising from the power relations between service users, carers and professionals. This is therefore a real opportunity for mentors to facilitate excellent reflection not only on how something should be done but also in the ethics and values underpinning the way it is done. In Chapter 4 we discuss some of the difficulties for mentors assessing qualities within the affective domain: this aspect of service user and carer involvement can be a fruitful area for exploring some of these key professional values. Indeed, some practice assessment documentation now includes elements of service user and carer feedback within the assessment process.

The complexities of managing busy caseloads and supporting learners is an added dimension to the context of practice learning. Many professions have embraced formal supervision to assist professionals to make sense of these complexities. Although the benefits of formal, individual supervision are accepted now, the inclusion of regular team, learning-focused opportunities for staff to discuss, plan and reflect on aspects of their professional life is also necessary. In the next case study Audrey Craig describes the efforts she has made to transform morning meetings into a more structured activity that can help those involved make sense of their practice and obtain support from their peers.

CASE STUDY

The benefits of a structured, learning-focused approach in a multi-professional morning meeting – Audrey Craig

In my role as manager of a Family Centre I hold responsibility for the provision of a professional service and the personal development of a team of seven practitioners. My own qualifications are in social work, while other team members hold a range of qualifications across a number of disciplines.

Ongoing studies by team members include undergraduate studies in health, pre-qualifying social work studies and postgraduate studies. The extent of professional experience varies widely. The team's primary function is to support families in their care of young children, acting on referrals from statutory agencies and self-referrals.

When I moved into my present post four years ago, from my perspective, team members appeared to lack structure within their working day, which in turn affected their work routines. There was also a lack of understanding of my professional accountability as the manager for team members' work. In short, I needed to know what was going on! As a clear response to these issues I introduced a formal daily morning meeting for all members of the team. This drew on my own earlier experiences of 'allocation meetings' in field social work and 'handovers' in residential child care. At that time my aims for the meeting were that it would be supportive and educative, that it would achieve better working relationships between team members, that it would provide a routine opportunity for a non-judgemental exchange of news and views, that it would lay the foundations for re-building a team ethos and that it would also be a forum for the socialisation of newer team members into suitable professional behaviours.

At first glance the morning meeting can be seen as simply a checking mechanism, recording that work undertaken the previous day has been achieved and that work planned for the forthcoming day has been properly allocated and planned. At a deeper level, as with one-to-one supervision, the morning meeting has three aspects or functions: administrative, educative and supportive (Kadushin, 2002). The administrative function can be seen as rather basic, covering areas such as annual leave and mileage claims; however, these aspects are all part of professional accountability. The meeting has established clear processes for key administrative tasks. While they can sound very dry these frameworks aim to keep practitioners and clients safe from drift and remind us all of our accountability to our various stakeholders.

The educative aspect of the meeting includes role modelling how professional discussions are conducted, in an application of social learning theory. Bandura (1977) contended that most behaviour was learned through observation. He argued this was how an individual formed ideas about what was expected and so served as a guide for action.

My role in conducting the meeting includes acting as a mentor to the team and my ambition is to follow Darling's (1984) definition of the characteristics of an effective mentor, namely to be an 'inspirer, investor and supporter'.

(Continued)

(Continued)

Accordingly the meeting is conducted in an encouraging and supportive style, with positive acknowledgements of the work achieved and encouragement for the tasks ahead. A considerable personal Investment is required on my part to achieve successful ways forward and the resolution of any disputes or differences in viewpoint.

The meeting is also a forum for team members to express any anxieties about their work and for these to be addressed. The responses to any concerns or anxieties can be emotional, practical or theory-based and can come from colleagues as well as their manager. One strength of the process is that it is collaborative and we are all involved. At their best, these conversations achieve reflection and learning about our work. Reflective practice is a constant theme in social work and I see it as the 'magic ingredient' which moves team members on from being competent to repeat tasks to being able to learn from them. To achieve not only single loop learning which takes place when goals, frameworks and approaches are taken for granted, but also double loop learning which involves questioning our underlying assumptions. So we ask, for example, 'What are our aims in this particular engagement with a family?' or 'Why do we practise as we do and what are the alternatives?'

Double loop questioning and learning helps us to plan in a reflective manner, taking into account earlier learning and 'practice wisdom' and theory. Through these discussions we sometimes build new understandings of our work as we examine the complexity of families' experiences and our roles in supporting them. At our best we sometimes approach transformative learning (Mezirow, 2000). Mezirow's theory of the mechanism of transformational learning includes three themes: experience, critical reflection and rational discourse. However, this process isn't smooth, as Mezirow also states that we do not make transformative changes if the material fits comfortably into what we already know (I would also add here 'what we think we know'). As our daily working reality often includes troubling new material and insights we are well placed to achieve significant professional and personal learning, but we must take the time to review our experiences and through the process of reflection and rational discourse learn to question our assumptions and be open to new meanings.

As in most areas of work SUN tends to be more beneficial than RAIN, especially when SUN equates to 'Suspend, Understand and Nurture' and RAIN equates to 'React, Assume and Insist' (Allan et al., 2002). Only on the basis of SUN can our morning meetings achieve their aims. This is always relevant particularly when we are joined by new team members who may arrive with basic skills and knowledge, unschooled in professional behaviours and attitudes. I have seen some great results from this approach with team members developing their skills not only in relation to their colleagues but also in relation to the children and parents they support.

Craig's case study is an effective reminder of the importance of supervision within professional practice. Howe (2008) voices his astonishment that so few social workers actually use supervision. He goes on to describe supervision as enabling practitioners to think about the emotional affect clients have on practitioners and the emotional affect practitioners can have on clients. Supervision can be the place where the complexities, joys and disappointments of professional practice can be examined. Inskipp and Proctor (1993), in their important work on supervision, identified three functions of supervision: the formative function (education); the restorative function (support); and the normative function (accountability). In her case study Craig identifies the potential threat apparent for some members of staff within the supervisory situation. Scaife (2010) discusses this and reflects on her own sense of vulnerability in a new practice setting, remembering that even the supervisor (mentor) appeared threatening. This is certainly possible when assessment is a function of the supervision, but the fear of being found out can also affect the relationship when there is no formal assessment element. It is vital for mentors to be cognisant of these potential fears and to think about the ways in which they can manage this situation. In Chapter 2 the importance of an effective relationship is discussed and the emphasis on the relationship is a key strategy for mentors to consider. Scaife (2010) offers 12 pointers to consider when establishing an effective supervision relationship, although these are just as useful within a mentoring context:

- create a climate of trust and safety;
- give one's full attention;
- provide containment;
- be prepared;
- bear in mind that people are trying to do their best;
- be prepared to exercise the authority that goes with the role of supervisor;
- recognise that the only concerns that can be successfully addressed are those owned or accepted by the supervisee;
- manage feedback thoughtfully;

- be prepared to show one's own practice and acknowledge one's imperfect practice;
- create and review the psychological context;
- agree the purpose of supervision and stay on track;
- agree on how to do supervision.

Howe considers reflection and supervision as essential elements for ensuring the 'emotionally intelligent, available and responsive social worker' (2008: 187). The same argument surely applies to all health and social care practitioners; indeed, Scaife (2010) suggests this is just as important for experienced practitioners as it is for students.

Chapter summary

Attempts such as this to support staff become increasingly necessary as health and social care practice and context change rapidly. Mentors need opportunities to make sense of these changes, particularly in relation to their support of students. If practice is chaotic then potentially learning can become chaotic. Mentors should remember that one of the key features about learning in practice is the unexpected and opportunistic nature of that learning; however, they are still required to manage and structure that learning. Without a framework or structure to practice learning there is a danger that learners will merely have a number of interesting experiences that are not transformed into meaningful learning. Effective mentors will help learners to make sense of these experiences despite the chaos and uncertainty that surround students. The requirement to continually develop skills and knowledge and critically reflect upon one's own practice is an important aspect of being a professional. The nature of practice learning can bring with it tensions and complexities, but when it is managed well it can also furnish learners with extraordinary learning opportunities.

Reflective activity

Now that you have read the chapter consider the activities below and reflect on the ways in which your own practice area deals with some of the issues surrounding the complexities of learning in a practice context:

- How do you ensure your practice remains contemporary?
- List the range of other professionals learners may be exposed to in your practice area.
- How do you currently incorporate service-user and carer involvement in your students' learning? Could you improve on this?
- What strategies do you use to help learners make sense of their practice experience?

References

Allan, D., Kingdom, M., Murmin, K. and Rudkin, D. (2002) *Sticky Wisdom: How to Start a Creative Revolution at Work.* Oxford: Wiley.

Bandura, A. (1977) *Social Learning Theory.* New York: General Learning Press.

Barr, H. and Sharland, E. (2012) 'Interprofessional education in qualifying social work'. In J. Lishman (ed.), *Social Work Education and Training.* London: Jessica Kingsley.

BBC (2010) 'Alcohol deaths up but overall drinking falls'. Available at http://news.bbc.co.uk/1/hi/health/845122.stm (last accessed 20 February 2011).

Clark, E. and Cox, C. (2011) 'Professional accountability'. In A. McIntosh, J. Gidman and E. Mason-Whitehead (eds), *Key Concepts in Healthcare Education.* London: Sage.

Commission for Social Care Inspection (2007) *Eight Principles for Involving Service Users and Carers.* London: CSCI.

Darling, L.A.W. (1984) 'What do nurses want in a mentor?', *Journal of Nursing Administration,* 14 (10): 42–44.

Department of Health (2000) *The NHS Plan: A Plan for Investment, A Plan for Reform.* London: HMSO.

Department of Health (2006) *Our Health, Our Care, Our Say: A New Direction for Community Services.* London: HMSO.

Gainsbury, S. (2010) 'Nurse mentors still "failing to fail" students'. Available at www.nursingtimes.net/whats-new-in-nursing/acute-care/nurse-mentors-still-failing-to-fail-students/5013926.article (last accessed 29 December 2011).

Galvani, S. and Forrester, D. (2008) *What works in training social workers about drug and alcohol use? A survey of student learning and readiness to practice. Final report for the Home Office.* Available at www.beds.ac.uk/departments/appliedsocialstudies/staff/sarah-galavani/galvani-forrester-horeport2008pdf (last accessed 14 February 2011).

General Social Care Council (2005) *Specialist Standards and Requirements for Post Qualifying Programmes: Children and Young People, Their Families and Carers.* London: GSCC.

Hammick, M., Freeth, D., Koppel, I., Reeves, S. and Barr, H. (2007) 'A best evidence systematic review of interprofessional education: *BEME Guide no. 9', Medical Teacher,* 29 (8): 735–751.

Health and Care Professions Council (2012) *Standards of Education and Training.* London: HCPC.

Howard, M.O., Allen-Meares, P. and Ruffolo, M.C. (2007) 'Teaching evidence-based practice: strategic and pedagogical recommendations for schools of social work', *Research on Social Work Practice,* 17 (5): 561–568.

Howe, D. (2008) *The Emotionally Intelligent Social Worker.* Basingstoke: Palgrave Macmillan.

Inskipp, F. and Proctor, B. (1993) *The Art, Craft and Tasks of Counselling Supervision. Part 1: Making the Most of Supervision.* Twickenham: Cascade.

Kadushin, A. (2002) *Supervision in Social Work* (4th edn). New York: Columbia University Press.

Knowles, M., Holton, E.F. and Swanson, R.A. (2005) *The Adult Learner: The Definitive Classic in Adult Education and Human Resource Development* (6th edn). Burlington, MA: Elsevier.

Marshall, M. and Gordon, F. (2005) 'Interprofessional mentorship: taking on the challenge', *Journal of Integrated Care,* 13 (2): 38–43.

McIntosh, A., Dulson, J. and Bailey-McHale, J. (2011) 'The value and values of service users'. In J. McCarthy and P. Rose (eds), *Values-based Health and Social Care.* London: Sage.

Mezirow, J. (2000) *Learning as Transformation: Critical Perspectives on a Theory in Progress.* San Francisco, CA: Jossey-Bass.

Nursing and Midwifery Council (2010) *Standards for Pre-Registration Nursing Education.* Available at http://standards.nmc-uk.org/PreReg Nursing/ statutory/background/Pages/Introduction.aspx (last accessed 27 March 2011).

Nutt, D.J., King, L.A. and Phillips, L.D. (2010) 'Drug harms in the UK: a multi criteria decision analysis', *The Lancet,* 376 (9752): 1558–1565.

Prime Minister's Commission on the Future of Nursing and Midwifery (2010) *Front Line Care: The Future of Nursing and Midwifery in England. Report of the Prime Minister's Commission on the Future of Nursing and Midwifery in England.* London: HMSO.

Sawyer, L. (2005) 'An outcomes based approach to domiciliary care', *Journal of Integrated Care,* 13 (3): 20–25.

Scaife, J. (2010) *Supervising the Reflective Practitioner: An Essential Guide to Theory and Practice.* Hove: Routledge.

Scriven, A. and Garman, S. (eds) (2005) *Promoting Health: Global Issues and Perspectives*. Basingstoke: Palgrave Macmillan.

Smith, P. and Sadler-Smith, E. (2006) *Learning in Organisations*. Oxford: Routledge.

St George's University of London (2009) *Drug related deaths in the UK – Annual Report 2009*. International Centre for Drug Policy available at www.sgul.ac.uk/about-st-georges/divisions/faculty-of-medicine-and-bio-medical-sciences/mental-health/icdp/webiste-pdfs/Executive%20sum-mary%20np-SAD%20AR%20209.pdf (last accessed 20 February 2011).

Stuart, C.C. (2007) *Assessment, Supervision and Support in Clinical Practice* (2nd edn). Edinburgh: Churchill Livingstone.

Tew, J., Gell, C. and Foster, S. (2004) *Learning From Experience: Involving Service Users and Carers in Mental Health Education and Training. Mental Health in Higher Education, National Institute for Mental Health in England (West Midlands)*. Nottingham: Trent Workforce Development Confederation.

The College of Social Work (2012*) Practice Educator Professional Standards for Social Work*. London: TCSW.

Walsh, C., Gordon, M., Marshall, M., Wilson, F. and Hunt, T. (2005) 'Interprofessional capability: a developing framework for interprofessional education', *Nurse Education in Practice*, 5 (4): 230–237.

Waters, B. (2001) 'Radical action for radical plans', *British Journal of Occupational Therapy*, 64 (11): 577–578.

World Health Organization (1998) *Health Promotion Glossary*. Geneva: WHO

Worsley, A. (2011) 'Interprofessional learning'. In A. MacIntosh, J. Gidman and E. Mason-Whitehead (eds), *Key Concepts in Healthcare Education*. London: Sage.

8 Evidence-based Practice

Case study: Claire Green

The provision and delivery of evidence-based care is a widely accepted model of service provision across health and social care. Contemporary health and social care practice is always dynamic; however, the recent pace of reforms and change has been relentless. The expectation that health and social care practitioners will engage in evidence-based practice in order to deliver safe, effective and quality care is ever more emphasised. Health and social care students are educationally prepared in relation to the skills required to deliver evidence-based practice; however, clearly the practice arena is where the application of these skills occurs. Mentors for health and social care students are in an ideal position to develop students' research skills and facilitate their ability to participate in evidence-based practice. The benefits of the mentor role modelling the delivery of evidence-based practice with consideration for patients' and clients' perspectives are potentially extensive in terms of students, the organisation, and the health and social care professions, as well as being vital to patients and clients.

This chapter will contextualise evidence-based practice within health and social care practice education and will consider key influences on the mentors' role within such practice. Evidence-based practice will be defined and the skills required by mentors will be examined in the context of the challenges presented by the reality of practice. The need to balance evidenced-based practice and values-based practice will also be considered.

The case study within this chapter is written by Claire Green who is a registered nurse working in an orthopaedic ward. Green gives an example of how some qualified professionals are fearful of further study despite the professional requirement that they engage in continuing professional development. She describes how mentorship can help these individuals overcome some of the perceived barriers to learning.

Chapter learning objectives

By the end of the chapter the reader should be able to:

- summarise what is meant by evidence-based practice;
- deconstruct the influences on the provision of evidence-based practice;
- critically evaluate the importance of the skills required by mentors in relation to evidence-based practice as well as the importance of these skills for students;
- judge the appropriateness of a range of strategies in order to facilitate the development of students' skills relating to evidence-based practice.

What is evidence-based practice?

The governance agenda embedded across health and social care has highlighted the demand and expectation for quality care underpinned by evidence-based practice. The importance of evidence-based practice for improving the quality and effectiveness of care has been articulated in government documents for several decades and reinforced in more recent legislation and policy (Darzi, 2008). Morango (2012) recognises the recent emphasis on evidence-based practice within social work, highlighting that social work based on research evidence is a cornerstone of the UK government's modernisation agenda for social services. The concept of evidence-based practice originated from medicine, with the evidence being predominantly quantitative and seen as scientific. Evidence-based practice is now a feature of all practice-based professions and it can be argued that evidence for best practice is gained from a broader range of sources. Common to definitions of evidence-based practice is that it is about making decisions regarding care, based on the integration of patients'/clients' values and needs, practitioners' experience and expertise, and the best available research findings. This recognition of patients'/clients' perspectives is crucial and reflects the philosophy that patients/clients should be involved in a meaningful way in their health and social care. The benefits of evidence-based practice are numerous and include improved patient outcomes, reduced costs, better standardisation in care and a reduction in the postcode lottery scenario, improved research skills for practitioners and higher quality care. Wallen et al. (2010) cite some of the outcomes of the evidence-based practice process as representing the formulation of practice protocols, standards and guidelines, all of which can lead to increased patient/client satisfaction due to improved outcomes which in turn improves satisfaction in health and social care organisations.

Skills required for evidence-based practice

Mentors are health and social care practitioners and as such have to draw on current research in order to remain professionally competent. Professional knowledge is expanding and practitioners need to be able to appraise the research relating to their area of practice; there are core skills and abilities that they will need in order to be confident and competent with the research process and the application of evidence based practice. Mentors and student mentors may find the following list useful when considering their own skills regarding understanding and implementing evidence-based practice:

- the ability to search for appropriate literature based on a question generated from practice, including the ability to apply literature searching skills across a range of databases;
- the ability to critically appraise the evidence for relevance and applicability, reliability and validity, and for cultural, ethnicity, ethical and gender appropriateness;
- the ability to synthesise and disseminate the findings to all relevant stakeholders, including patients/clients, and then implement the evidence into practice in a timely manner;
- the ability to contribute to or initiate the development of policy, guidelines and procedures;

- the ability to evaluate the impact of evidence introduced into the practice arena including gaining patient/client feedback, and make changes based on the analysis of evaluation;
- the confidence to deliver presentations to team members and senior members of the organisation, as well as at conferences;
- the confidence to write for publication, for example sharing experiences related to the impact of evidence on patient/client care;
- the confidence to participate in practice development and research and role model their research skills to students.

Chapter link

See Chapter 2 for a further discussion of role modelling.

Role modelling is a key and powerful aspect of the mentor's role. Gopee (2010) suggests that mentors should embody the qualities of an evidence-based practitioner and be able to adopt changes and adaptations in interventions that will benefit the health of patients and service users and this is a characteristic that students can emulate. Within social work, Morango (2012) highlights a mentor's responsibility to role model evidence-based practice, identifying that with increased education social work mentors are more able to:

- demonstrate and apply the principles of evidence-based practice in their day-to-day professional practice;
- disseminate and share their skills and knowledge relating to evidence-based practice to colleagues and the professional arena in which they are based;
- facilitate social work students to practise evidence-based practice in their placements.

In the following case study Claire Green identifies barriers that can potentially hinder professionals in relation to their ongoing professional development which may then have a detrimental effect on their ability to engage in evidence-based practice.

Evidence-based practice – Claire Green

Lifelong learning is the concept that 'it's never too soon or late for learning', a philosophy that has taken root in a host of organisations, including the National Health Service. In the healthcare setting lifelong learning is about growth and opportunity, envisaged to make sure that both staff and the organisations they work in can acquire new knowledge and skills in order to both realise individual potential and to help shape and change things for the future. Despite the increased duration of primary, secondary and higher education, the knowledge and skills gained by individuals are not usually sufficient for a professional career which can span decades. One of the reasons that lifelong education has become so crucial is the acceleration of scientific and technological progress that is clearly relevant in all areas of nursing.

The Nursing and Midwifery Council (2008) requires nurses to keep their knowledge and skills up to date and participate in learning activities (currently thirty-five hours of study over the previous three years). Bahn (2007) has identified three reasons why nurses engage in post-registration learning: these are described as personal, academic and vocational. Beder (1989) also identified a personal orientation towards learning as the seeking of personal growth and development. Academic learning embodies the theoretical, evidence-based knowledge sought by the profession, and vocational learning involves the acquisition of knowledge in a material sense, namely to be able to perform specialised tasks adequately and safely (Cust, 1996).

There are, however, many barriers which can stop nurses accessing learning opportunities. Extrinsic barriers include inequitable access to flexible programmes and a lack of funding, institutional attitudes and inflexible working practices (Buchan and Secombe, 2004). There are also internal barriers which can prevent a nurse accessing learning opportunities, one of which is fear of the unknown (Cooley, 2008). While there has been a prolific development of distance and e-learning opportunities, and while these can provide a rich and flexible learning environment, Cook et al. (2004) suggest that systems failure and a lack of contact can cause stress and anxiety. Another intrinsic barrier to learning is the guilt that some nurses feel about possibly neglecting family commitments.

Sharon (pseudonym) is a staff nurse on an orthopaedic/trauma ward in a general hospital who undertook her nurse training during the 1980s and has not completed any formal education since then. A recently appointed ward manager has told Sharon that she must now undertake a module from the courses offered by her employer. Her attitude towards this is negative and she exhibits fear, guilt and complacency. Her fear is shown by the statement 'I'm just not academic, and I don't do computers'. Bahn (2007) suggests this attitude is not uncommon in nurses who completed their training before 2000. Sharon's guilt is vocalised when she says 'I've got children at home to look after'. Cooley (2008) argues that adults and children can do their homework together: in this way Sharon's children would begin to see studying as a positive use of their time. Her complacency is also demonstrated when she says 'I just want to do my job, go home and get paid each month'. This demonstrates that Sharon's practice does not necessarily take into account the latest research. Evidence-based practice encompasses integrating the best research with clinical expertise and patient values in order to facilitate decision making and provide quality care. For nurses to achieve this, they must first be aware of what the current evidence shows rather than relying on old methods that have since been updated.

Mentorship has been defined in many different ways, but perhaps the simplest definition has come from Jarvis (1995) who states that the mentor–student relationship should have the explicit purpose of helping another individual to learn. While the concept of mentorship is usually associated with student or newly qualified nurses, Northcott (2000) identifies that even experienced practitioners will benefit from having a mentor at various points during their career. In Sharon's case she would benefit from having a mentor to help her to identify specific learning needs and break down some of the barriers that are stopping her from accessing education. Sharon's fear could be addressed by enrolling her on a Return to Study course, offered free-of-charge by her employer, where she could meet others in a similar position to herself; this would help give her a sense of belonging, something which Santy (2006) identifies as a factor in readiness to learn. Nurses state that they want to improve the care they deliver, and here the mentor's role could be to involve Sharon in searching for appropriate evidence and guidelines, thus ensuring that the care she gives is based on current best practice guidelines.

An individual nurse is accountable for the care they deliver (NMC, 2008). The NMC makes continuing professional development mandatory for nurses through PREP, although there is little evidence that standards are being met. Sharon fulfils her PREP requirement by completing her annual mandatory training. While it could be argued that she is indeed meeting the professional standards that are required of her, it can also be seen that she does not deliver best quality care as she

(Continued)

(Continued)

is continuing to use methods which she was taught twenty-five years previously, even when she knows that further training has been available during this time. The NMC could also adopt a more rigorous and robust attitude to PREP as currently this is self-regulated by individual nurses. E-mail correspondence between the author and the NMC (August 2009) reveals that in 2006 the NMC made the decision not to request details on how nurses met their PREP requirements, and to only request this information if another area of a nurse's practice was called into question.

To conclude the author would recommend a learning mentor in all health care settings in order to identify the learning needs of both staff and the organisations in which they work and to enable standards of care to rise. This would ensure that those nurses who currently may have issues regarding their readiness to engage in formal learning could be supported; this in turn would ultimately improve standards of care in practice.

Barriers to evidence-based practice

Despite the importance and value of evidence-based practice being advocated by government, health and social care professional bodies, health and social care professional education curricula, and patient, client and service user groups, there are still a number of concerns regarding a lack of consistency in its implementation. Within social work Mullen et al. (2005) have asserted that limited numbers of social workers are adopting evidence-based approaches to their practice. When considering evidence-based practice within nursing, Taylor and Allen (2007) highlight the limited extent to which practice is based on evidence. Flores-Mateo and Argimon (2007) identified that a consistent finding of health care research is the gap between best evidence-based practice and actual clinical care: they argue that between 10 and 40 per cent of patients do not receive evidence-based care in relation to clinical guidelines. Caldwell et al. (2006) assert that there are multi-factorial and complex challenges intrinsic to implementing evidence-based practice. Wallen et al. (2010) agree with this, suggesting that, despite many government reports, an educational focus and consumer expectations the integration of evidence-based practice into day-to-day practice is not consistent and the gap between practice and research is still significant. Some of the key barriers impacting on health and social care professionals' ability to engage in evidence-based practice are presented below:

- a lack of confidence in research skills;
- time constraints;
- inaccessibility of research evidence;
- a lack of confidence in the organisation to support evidence-based practice;
- a lack of confidence in information technology skills;
- a lack of appropriateness of research findings for practice;
- a lack of resources including administrative;
- a lack of research mentors.

Work undertaken by Webster et al. (2003) regarding nurses' research skills identified that only a third of nurses in the sample group used computers to regularly access evidenced resources. A significant proportion of these nurses, over 30 per cent, believed that searching for evidence was an ineffective use of time which detracted from patient care and that evidence should lie within accessible care pathways and policies. In relation to a lack of confidence in research skills, Pagoto et al. (2007) argue that health care students tend to be taught the research process as opposed to how to use research in delivering best practice. Nagy et al. (2001) suggest that a barrier to the integration of evidence in decision making in the practice setting was that research findings lacked applicability and clinical credence. All of the potential barriers above have implications for mentors in relation both to their own research activity and to nurturing student research skills.

Health and social care professionals need to be supported by their organisation in research endeavours. An identified potential barrier is the perception that the organisation does not always support such an engagement in research activity. Registered health professionals in research undertaken by Moore et al. (2012) reported that a research culture was not embedded within the organisation, and they identified several barriers including:

- there were no formal frameworks to support innovation;
- staff perceived that they lacked the capacity to incorporate research activity into their day-to-day practice;
- there was no clearly articulated financial support to allow staff the time to innovate or any provision to cover leave for staff development;
- the organisation did not appear to reward innovation.

Mentors may have access to local research/practice development units or will form partnerships, for example with local universities, in order to gain support for their research endeavours. It is, however, of paramount importance that a strong infrastructure exists within the organisation, in order to support and sustain evidence-based practice, practice development and other research activities.

Chapter link

Go to Chapter 9 to review the concept of leadership within mentorship.

One initiative that has the potential to foster evidence-based practice is the introduction of education governance into health and social care organisations. The NHS North West Workforce and Education Directorate (2009) have produced a guidance document to facilitate a strategy for education governance and have also pledged to support other NHS organisations in establishing education governance. The document cites many principles and benefits of education governance, including that:

- education governance has the same priority as clinical governance;
- there is a multi-professional governance approach, with enhanced learning leadership, thus enabling best practice to be shared across all health care disciplines and across all levels of staff involved in the delivery of health services;
- the quality of health care education and learning is improved continuously in the context of its importance in improving the quality of patient care;
- there is effective partnership working across placement and education providers and specifically between employers and education to inform the planning, delivery and assessment of education in practice and academic settings. (NHS North West Workforce and Education Directorate, 2009: 5)

It appears that the crucial benefit of education governance is an improvement in the quality of care for patients, clients and service users. It can be argued that the introduction of education governance principles will invariably improve the learning culture and environment and so foster further engagement in evidence-based practice. Health and social care mentors should consider the extent to which the principles of education governance exist within their organisation and how they can use their leadership skills to influence a more explicit recognition of education governance. Considering the issues identified in Green's case study, it is interesting to consider the extent to which fully embedded education governance would address barriers to learning and best evidence for best practice.

Strategies to enhance evidence-based practice

It is vital for mentors to consider how they can facilitate evidence-based practice both in relation to themselves and in relation to their students. Mentors may not be undertaking empirical research in order to generate evidence for practice; however, they should be critical and informed consumers of research. This effective consumption of research is no less important than undertaking research and is in fact necessary for students to observe the skilled appraisal and application of good evidence within a practice setting. In terms of their appraisal skills mentors need to consider what constitutes appropriate evidence. We mentioned earlier in the chapter that evidence-based practice has its roots in scientific, positivist approaches that usually generate quantitative data. Within healthcare randomised controlled trials that produce quantitative information are seen as the gold standard of evidence. It can be argued that with health and social care provision being ever more scrutinised in terms of cost efficacy there is an increased emphasis on what Burton and Chapman (2004) describe as the orthodox approach to evidence-based practice. They describe this approach as research on the relationship between practices and outcomes, with the focus on practitioners undertaking practice that is known to be effective. Although obviously a recognised and accepted approach, this does not take account of patients'/clients' views, values, beliefs, experiences and preferences, as well as practitioners' expertise. Goding and Edwards (2002) suggest that evidence-based practice de-emphasises practice experience and intuition. Contemporary health and social care practice strives for a patient/client centrality in service provision and adopts a holistic approach to practice. Burton and Chapman (2004: 18) assert that whilst evidence-based practice does acknowledge clinical judgement to some extent, this is not well developed. They suggest that practitioners gain their evidence from a range of sources, including:

- experience;
- values, beliefs and attitudes;
- an appraisal of the current situation;
- theory;

- knowledge from multiple sources, including service user feedback, personal, scientific, craft and interpersonal;
- imperatives, including personal, interpersonal, organisational, professional, legal and governmental;
- judgement which draws on the above facets and integrates them.

In order to ensure a balance between evidence-based care and values-based care, mentors could consider the adoption of a bricoleur approach to research activity. Warne and McAndrew (2009) describe bricolage as a multifaceted approach to sourcing evidence which includes the lived experience of patients/clients. They explain that by adopting a bricolage approach, practitioners will avoid the development of limited reductionist, monological forms of knowledge that disregards context. They also assert that by harnessing practitioners' personal knowledge and the patient/client experience, genuine patient/client-centred care can be facilitated. The context in which care is delivered presents the application of traditional evidence-based practice with some difficulties. Burton and Chapman (2004) describe the health and social care environment as complex and multifactorial, an 'open system' that is subject to unpredictable and multiple influences as opposed to being enclosed and controlled. It can be argued that an enclosed and controlled environment would be more congruent with quantitative methods of underpinning evidence-based practice; however, this is not the reality of practice. An example of a naturalistic approach to underpinning evidence for health and social care practice is the use of narrative inquiry. Hardy et al. (2009) suggest that through the use of narrative-based approaches to health care inquiry, practitioners can have their eyes and ears opened by the information gained from their daily discussions with service users. It is clear that health and social care professional practitioners need evidence for practice that is appropriately situated and contextual. Mentors must consider the range of evidence that they are appraising, and through the adoption of a bricolage approach can balance positivist approaches to evidence-based practice with practitioner and patient/client-centred evidence. By role modelling this approach, in particular through the identification of a wide range of credible evidence, the mentor will facilitate the students' development of research knowledge as well as reducing barriers to the students' research potential.

Chapter link

See Chapter 3 for a further discussion of ways to facilitate learning and Chapter 6 for a discussion concerning the learning environment.

A further strategy for mentors to employ in developing students' evidence-based practice skills is the development of critical thinking skills. Standards for pre-qualifying professional educational programmes clearly articulate the expectation that students should be engaged in evidence-based practice. However, in nursing Bradbury-Jones et al. (2011) highlight concerns regarding newly qualified nurses' critical thinking ability. Mentors can influence both students' skills in critical thinking and foster critical thinking in the team, thus influencing the learning environment. Myrick and Yonge (2001) identified the major role mentors have in influencing the practice setting and the degree of support students can receive from mentors and others in the learning environment. If the mentor–student relationship is effective a student will feel able to discuss and explore issues with their mentor and to ask the naïve questions that often facilitate deep learning. In turn the mentor will encourage this exploration and provoke challenging questions in order to develop their own critical thinking skills as well as those of the student. For mentors considering the nature of critical thinking for evidence-based practice Aveyard et al. (2011) highlight the core critical thinking skills as interpretation, analysis, inference, evaluation, explanation and self-regulation, and offer the following useful explanations:

- critical thinking – this is where you adopt a questioning and thoughtful approach to what you see, hear or read, rather than accepting information at face value;
- critical analysis – this is where you break down or explore in depth all the available information relating to a practice question or issue. This may involve exploring what is happening and the reasons for this. You will need to access alternative perspectives, including theory;
- critical appraisal – this is where you consider the strengths and limitations of each piece of evidence.

In Table 8.1 Aveyard and Sharp (2011) have suggested various ideas to help mentors role model an evidence-based approach.

As well as encouraging and developing critical thinking in students, mentors need to make judgements regarding students' competence with evidence-based practice. Ilic (2009) highlights how difficult it is to assess competence in evidence-based practice and suggests the use of a diary where a student will record activities related to research and evidence-based practice, for example evidence of literature searches or critical appraisals. As well as use of a diary a mentor can observe and question a student regarding evidence-based practice and encourage them to explore evidence from a range of sources with a focus on patient/client experience.

Table 8.1   Role modelling critical thinking skills in professional practice
(adapted from work by Aveyard and Sharp (2011))

Ways to role model critical thinking within professional practice	Benefits of these approaches
• demonstrate core critical thinking skills in daily practice; • be clear, articulate and explicit about decision making and the uncertainty of practice; • identify, question and critique sources of information; • reflect openly on own practice; • encourage critical reflection on practice by students and colleagues; • ask questions, including higher level questions, of self and student to encourage critical thinking; • explore alternative perspectives; • present arguments and counter arguments; • critically reflect on own realities of practice.	• theory and practice application would be enhanced; • critical thinking skills would be practised and developed; • students would recognise what was expected of them; • the evidence for practice would be more explicit, facilitating accountability; • team members would become socialised into thinking critically and would recognise the benefits; • the learning environment would be enhanced; • improved patient/client care and outcomes.

Mentors and student mentors should consider opportunities for becoming involved in research either as research participants or researchers. This active involvement in the research process will maximise learning beyond the effective consumption, appraisal and application of evidence to practice. By utilising partnership links, mentors of health and social care students can also identify potential research studies that may be appropriate for students to take part in as participants. Within research undertaken by Bradbury-Jones et al. (2011), students who experienced being research participants cited several benefits, including a strengthening of the self, a strengthening of knowledge and a strengthening of clinical practice. Furthermore, some students identified that they had become sufficiently motivated to engage in research when they became a registered professional. If health and social care students become involved in research it is vital that mentors support these students throughout the process. Lev et al. (2010) emphasise the importance of good mentorship for mentees undertaking research in order to increase the research self-efficacy of students.

A further strategy to enhance evidence-based practice is interprofessional mentorship. The benefits of interprofessional learning have been well established. Interprofessional mentorship already occurs on an informal basis in that students on a professional education programme will spend time with professionals from different disciplines within health and social care. This time tends to be mainly observational and on a visit basis. With changes made by the NMC (2010) to the due regard principle, nursing placements can now incorporate other professionals within the mentorship and assessment features of the student placement circuit. Marshall and Gordon (2005) define interprofessional mentorship as occasions when a health or social care professional facilitates, supervises and assesses students in a practice setting. The value of interprofessional mentorship to evidence-based practice is that students will be exposed to a wider range of evidence and different approaches to care delivery. It can be argued that this will facilitate students' appreciation of a wider range of alternative perspectives, including those of patients/clients and service users. Ultimately this should facilitate the development of interprofessional learning and evidence within a range of health and social care practice environments.

Chapter link

See Chapter 7 for a further discussion of interprofessional mentorship and assessment.

Chapter summary

The expectation and value of evidence-based practice are clearly articulated by the United Kingdom government through the quality and governance agenda. Evidence-based practice is embedded within the aims of health and social care organisations; however, there appears to be several barriers to its implementation at the practice level. Registered health and social care professionals need to be critical consumers of research and undertake a range of research activities. It is therefore vital that mentors consider their own skills relating to evidence-based practice and practice development as well as researchers. It is particularly important for mentors to utilise their leadership skills to influence educational governance and colleagues in order to enhance the application of evidence-based practice across practice settings. Mentors need to reflect on their own approach to evidence-based practice, with the goal of facilitating students to adopt a balanced approach where evidence-based care is harmonised with values-based care.

Reflective activity

Having read the chapter you should be able to give more consideration to your skills and your approach to evidence-based practice. Think about the questions below in the context of evidence-based practice within your role as mentor:

- How would you evaluate your skills relating to evidence-based practice?
- What is the approach to evidence-based practice within your team?
- Do you encounter any barriers regarding the implementation of evidence-based practice?
- If so, what strategies do you and your team employ to address these barriers?
- Are you aware of governance in relation to education in your organisation?
- In what ways do you and your team ensure a balance between values-based practice and evidence-based practice?
- In what ways could you seek opportunities for yourself, colleagues and students to engage in research either as participants or researchers?

References

Aveyard, H. and Sharp, P. (2011) *Are we modelling an evidenced based, critical approach within nurse education and practice?* Available at www.rcn.org.uk/__data/assets/pdf_file/0005/433526/Are_we_modelling_an_evidence_based.pdf (last accessed 24 June 2011).

Aveyard, H., Sharp, P. and Woolliams, M. (2011) *A Beginners Guide to Critical Thinking and Writing in Health and Social Care.* Maidenhead: Open University Press.

Bahn, D. (2007) 'Reasons for post registration learning: impact of the learning experience', *Nurse Education Today,* 27: 715–722.

Beder, H. (1989) 'Purposes and philosophies of adult education'. In S. Merriam and P. Cunningham (eds), *Handbook of Adult and Continuing Education.* London: Jossey-Bass.

Bradbury-Jones, C., Stewart, S., Irvine, F. and Sambrook, S. (2011) 'Nursing students' experiences of being a research participant: findings from a longitudinal study', *Nurse Education Today*, 31: 107–111.

Buchan, J. and Secombe, I. (2004) *Fragile Future: A Review of the UK Nursing Labour Market Review*. London: Royal College of Nursing.

Burton, M. and Chapman, M. (2004) 'Problems of evidence based practice in community based services', *Journal of Learning Disabilities*, 8 (1): 1–35.

Caldwell, K., Coleman, K., Copp, G., Bell, L. and Ghazi, F. (2006) 'Preparing for professional practice: how well does professional training equip health and social care practitioners to engage in evidenced-based practice?', *Nurse Education Today*, 27: 518–528.

Cook, G., Thynne, E., Weatherhead, E., Glenn, S., Mitchell, A. and Bailey, P. (2004) 'Distance learning in post-qualifying nurse education', *Nurse Education Today*, 24: 269–276.

Cooley, M. (2008) 'Nurses' motivations for studying third level post-registration nursing programmes and the effects of studying on their personal and work lives', *Nurse Education Today*, 28: 588–594.

Cust, J. (1996) 'A relational view of learning: implications for nurse education', *Nurse Education Today*, 16 (4): 256–262.

Darzi, A. (2008) *High Quality Care for All: NHS Next Stage Final Review*. London: DH.

Flores-Mateo, G. and Argimon, J. (2007) 'Evidence based practice in postgraduate health care: a systematic review', *BCM Health Services Research*, 7 (119): 1–26.

Goding, L. and Edwards, K. (2002) 'Evidence based practice', *Nurse Researcher*, 9 (4): 45–57.

Gopee, N. (2010) *Practice Teaching in Healthcare*. London: Sage.

Hardy, S., Gregory, S. and Ramjeet, J. (2009) 'An exploration of intent for narrative methods of inquiry', *Researcher*, 16 (4): 7–19.

Ilic, D. (2009) 'Assessing competence in Evidenced Based Practice: strengths and limitations of current tools in practice', *BCM Medical Education*, 9 (53): 1–5.

Jarvis, P. (1995) 'Towards a philosophical understanding of mentoring', *Nurse Education Today*, 15: 414–419.

Lev, E., Kolassa, J. and Bakken, L. (2010) 'Faculty mentors' and students' perceptions of students' research self-efficacy', *Nurse Education Today*, 30: 169–174.

Marshall, M. and Gordon, F. (2005) 'Interprofessional mentorship: taking on the challenge', *Journal of Integrated Care*, 13 (2): 38–43.

Moore, J., Crozier, K. and Kite, K. (2012) 'An action research approach for developing research and innovation in nursing and midwifery practice: building research capacity in one NHS foundation trust', *Nurse Education Today*, 32: 39–45.

Morango, P. (2012) 'Evaluation of social work education'. In J. Lishman (ed.), *Social Work Education and Training*. London: Jessica Kingsley.

Mullen, E., Shlonsky, A., Bledsoe, S. and Bellamy, J. (2005) 'From concept to implementation: challenges facing evidence based social work', *Evidence and Policy: A Journal of Research, Debate and Practice,* 1 (1): 61–84.

Myrick, F. and Yonge, O. (2001) 'Creating a climate for critical thinking in the preceptorship experience', *Nurse Education Today,* 21: 461–467.

Nagy, S., Lumby, J., McKinley, S. and Macfarlane, C. (2001) 'Nurses' beliefs about the conditions that hinder or support evidence-based nursing', *International Journal of Nursing Practice,* 7 (5): 314–321.

National Health Service North West (2009) *Making Education Governance a Reality in the North West*. Manchester: NHS North West's Workforce and Education Directorate.

Northcott, N. (2000) 'Mentorship in nursing', *Nursing Management,* 7 (3): 30–32.

Nursing and Midwifery Council (2008) *The PREP Handbook*. London: NMC.

Nursing and Midwifery Council (2010) *Standards for Pre-registration Nursing Education*. London: NMC.

Pagoto, S., Spring, B., Coups, E., Mulvaney, S., Coutu, M. and Ozakinci, G. (2007) 'Barriers and facilitators of evidence based practice perceived by behavioural science health professionals', *Journal of Clinical Psychology,* 63 (7): 695–705.

Santy, J. (2006) 'Scaling the castle walls: bringing orthopaedic and trauma nurses together online'. Presentation at RCN Society of Orthopaedic & Trauma Nursing's Sands of Time: Orthopaedic & Trauma Nursing, Past Present & Future Conference, 14–15 September.

Taylor, S. and Allen, D. (2007) 'Visions of evidence-based nursing practice', *Nurse Researcher,* 15 (1): 78–83.

Wallen, G., Mitchell, S., Melnyk, B., Fineout-Overholt, E, Miller-Davies, C., Yates, J. and Hastings, C. (2010) 'Implementing evidence-based practice: effectiveness of a structured multifactorial mentorship programme', *Journal of Advanced Nursing,* 66 (12): 2761–2771.

Warne, T. and McAndrew, S. (2009) 'Constructing a bricolage of nursing research, education and practice', *Nurse Education Today,* 29: 855–858.

Webster, J., Davies, J., Holt, V., Stallan, G., News, K. and Yegdich, T. (2003) 'Australian nurses' and midwives' knowledge of computers and their attitudes to using them in practice', *Journal of Advanced Nursing,* 41 (2): 140–146.

9   Leadership

Case studies: Julie Hatton and John Davison

All health and social care professionals have the potential to act as leaders in several aspects of their role. Some leaders will be high profile, introducing the major changes that will redesign or improve service delivery or taking the lead in a crisis or complex situations. However, most leadership occurs within everyday health and social care practice with professionals endeavouring to provide quality care. The expectation that health and social care professionals will possess and utilise leadership skills at the fundamental interface of practice is reflected in professional and regulatory bodies' codes of conduct. Definitions of a leader will depend on the context, but a common element of most definitions and explanations of what makes someone a leader is that they should have the ability to motivate and influence others to achieve positive goals that will enhance the effectiveness of organisations, teams and individuals and ultimately improve client/patient care. Mentors for health and social care students are in the privileged position of being able to influence those students and as such are key leaders of learning within health and social care practice education. From reviewing previous chapters in this book, it is evident that via their mentorship role mentors can build on their existing leadership skills and that many of the skills they require for quality mentorship are congruent with those necessary for leadership. Every mentor, as well as developing their own leadership skills within practice and within their mentorship role, will also have responsibility for leading students' practice education experience and identifying and fostering their potential for leadership. It is important for students that their mentors lead that practice experience by maximising learning opportunities and facilitating professional and personal development.

This chapter will contextualise leadership within the mentorship role with due consideration for the skills required to lead practice education and each student's individual practice learning experience. The influence of leadership on learning in a broad sense will also be considered. Students have reported that it is vital for mentors to possess leadership qualities. The attributes that mentors require in order to be effective leaders will thus be examined along with relevant approaches to and styles of leadership.

The first case study author, Julie Hatton, a social worker, works in social services as a manager of residential services for adults with learning disabilities. Hatton identifies that core skills are intrinsic to the role of a manager, a leader, and a mentor. She highlights some of the positive benefits to staff of having access to a mentor/leader; however, she also discusses the tension between her role as a manager, a mentor and a leader of staff members.

The second case study author is John Davison, a district nursing specialist practitioner and team leader within adult community nursing services. Davison asserts the importance of mentors developing students into future leaders and discusses the value of participative and transformational theories of leadership for mentors. As with the first case study author, Davison also identifies the similarities between leadership and mentorship qualities.

The expectation for mentors to possess and enact leadership qualities in relation to both patient/client care and practice learning is clearly articulated in health and social care professional education curricula, professional codes of conduct and job specifications. The ability to realise this expectation requires highly skilled mentors who can influence the learning culture of the organisation, their team and their students. Health and social care professionals are not automatically leaders by virtue of their profession; however, they can learn and develop the skills that are necessary for leadership. Therefore this chapter will consider those skills and the development of these in relation to key aspects that are identified within the presented case studies.

Chapter learning outcomes

By the end of the chapter the reader should be able to:

- summarise the key features of effective leadership;
- critically reflect on their leadership skills in relation to both students' practice education placements and the learning environment;
- evaluate the strategies they use in order to develop students' leadership potential.

Leadership and mentorship

Health and social care professionals practising within the current challenging political and economic landscape need to employ skills of problem solving, critical thinking and team working, including working across boundaries and reflective practice. They must also take leading roles within complex and diverse health and social care practice arenas, utilising highly developed interpersonal skills in order to articulate their contributions both to the organisation and their profession. Leadership is embedded as a key concept within contemporary health and social care and is reflected in codes of conduct for registered professionals (Nursing and Midwifery Council [NMC], 2008a, 2008b; Health and Care Profession's Council [HCPC], 2012) as well as in standards of education for pre-registration educational programmes for pre-qualifying students (NMC, 2010; HCPC, 2012; The College of Social Work [TCSW], 2012). Health and social care professionals occupy a leadership role in several aspects of their practice, including leading the team or initiatives when particular professional interest and expertise is appropriate, employing leadership within mentorship and leading on their own continuing professional development. Schira (2007) also highlights how professionals lead with patients/clients and families by virtue of their professional knowledge and skills. The recognition that all registered professionals have a leadership role is a shift away from the traditional view of leaders as individuals in senior and often management positions. Stanley (2008) argues that within nursing the terms 'nursing leadership' and 'nursing management' are often used as interchangeable concepts despite being clearly different, with literature and research often being developed in order to inform those in management positions, thereby leading to an acceptance that insights gained from management literature are transferable to leadership. Given the notion that leadership and management are different concepts then health and social care professionals need to seek out appropriate literature and evidence to support their leadership roles. While a manager may also lead the roles are not necessarily analogous, whereas mentorship and leadership are inextricably linked.

Most health and social care professionals will at times need to mentor and lead another's learning in some capacity, for example with a new or junior member of staff, and will certainly need to lead their own learning. Conway (2007) posits that all developmental experiences, including mentorship and formal learning, are essential for developing leadership skills and should be seen as leadership activities in themselves. When discussing the leadership role of qualified mentors, Kinnel and Hughes (2010) highlight how the value of being an effective leader is consistent with the value of receiving recognition and respect for committing to ensuring that health care students experience quality practice placements, stating that 'Leadership is an integrated role that mentors have to undertake whilst also executing their mentorship skills' (2010: 194). The congruency between mentorship and leadership is explicit, with many mentor responsibilities being consistent with leadership skills and behaviours. Key aspects of a mentor's role, such as relationship building, teaching, supporting and guiding the student's personal and professional development, being competent in practice, influencing others in relation to the learning environment and role modelling, are also fundamental to leadership. Zilembo and Monterosso (2008) suggest that leadership is all about relationships encompassing influence and vision and the embracement of the professional values of the leader and the organisation. Mentors for health and social care students are likely to recognise their role as having a positive influence on their students in terms of professional values and practice; however, they may not recognise or describe themselves as leaders due to the integral nature of leadership within their role. Vance (2002) asserts that the connection between mentorship and leadership is strong and identifies core functions of both roles. These functions, presented below, may help mentors to more explicitly recognise their existing leadership skills. Vance (2002) argues that mentors/leaders:

- energise;
- motivate;
- create change in individuals, teams and organisations;
- are role models;
- are teachers;
- are professional guides;
- are advocates and counsellors.

Chapter link

Think about the ways in which your practice demonstrates mastery. (See Chapter 1 for a further discussion.)

Students have reported the importance of their mentors possessing leadership skills, with Allan et al. (2008) finding that students perceived mentors who displayed positive and transformational leadership skills as actually enhancing the practice learning environment. Health and social care students regularly cite practice competence and expertise as being a desirable attribute for their mentors to have. This aspect is a further connection with leadership, as practice leadership is rooted in practice competence and expertise. The authors of this book assert that mentorship is an advanced professional activity as outlined by the Quality Assurance Agency. Frameworks that articulate the level of practice required for advanced practice or advanced professional activity tend to incorporate both mentorship and leadership skills along with other required skills. The following is an example taken from an advanced practice portfolio devised by the National Leadership and Innovation Agency for Healthcare, NHS Wales (2010), which suggests areas for professionals to collate evidence pertaining to leadership and education/leadership.

Table 9.1   Examples of skills required for advanced practice

Leadership	Education
• identifying the need for change, leading and managing innovation including service development; • networking; • developing a case for change; • team development; • negotiation and influencing skills.	• principles of teaching and learning; • creating and contributing to a positive learning environment; • supporting others to develop knowledge and skills; • mentorship, teaching and coaching; • service user/carer teaching.

What is clear from the examples above is the transferability across and commonality between mentorship and leadership. The importance of leadership within mentorship is asserted by the NMC (2008) and is part of mentorship preparation educational programmes for social workers, health professionals and nurses. The authors of this book are part of a core team of lecturers who deliver mentorship preparation programmes and it is interesting to consider the academic assignment set for the module. Part of this is to develop an innovation in practice which facilitates teaching and learning. The student mentors are required to introduce their innovation, which as well as enhancing student learning contributes to the learning environment and often involves a service change that will have a positive effect on client/patient care. This serves to demonstrate the utilisation of mentorship and leadership skills and qualities within the mentor role. The positive influence of leadership on practice learning is evident here. Mentors should consider their existing leadership skills and how to utilise them effectively and also look at their development as a leader in the context of leadership approaches and styles, characteristics and behaviours. In the following case study Hatton identifies that while there are some similarities between mentorship/leadership and management, it is still a challenge to mentor staff that she must manage and may have to enact disciplinary processes with. Hatton concludes that while some aspects of mentorship/leadership are useful for supervision and for facilitating the continuing professional development of staff, it is inappropriate for managers to mentor staff in the fullest sense of the concept of mentorship.

Leadership – Julie Hatton

I am the manager of a residential service for adults with learning disabilities. I believe it is inherent in that role to offer leadership and to support the development opportunities of those I manage. I became interested in exploring the complexities associated with a line manager mentoring those who they also manage. I wanted to identify the tensions in such relationships, the potential positive and/or negative outcomes for the mentee, the mentor and the wider organisation. Lewis (1996) has suggested that the mentoring relationship involves a set of processes in which a mentor offers help, guidance, advice and support in order to facilitate learning and development in a mentee. On further research it became apparent that mentoring falls into two broad types (Aldred et al., 2008). These categories have been described as developmental mentoring (supporting the mentee's learning/development) and sponsorship mentoring (seen as fast tracking mentees in their careers). It would appear that the common thread within both of these mentoring types is the relationship between mentor and mentee (Lewis, 1996; Foster-Turner, 2006; Aldred et al., 2008). Key to these relationships are the skills that the mentor brings: these skills have been described by the Lewis (1996), General Social Care Council (GSCC) (2002a), Aldred et al. (2008) and Ali and Panther (2008), and include being open and honest in communication, empathetic, and having and being willing to share knowledge and expertise.

It is interesting to consider if any of the mentor's skills dovetail with those identified as key skills for management and leadership roles. Mullins (1990) described management as the ability to get things done by using other people to achieve stated organisational goals. In contrast leadership is defined by Hannagan (1998) as the process of achieving specific goals through the ability to motivate others. The most effective managers will have some if not all of the qualities associated with effective leadership skills. Huckabee and Wheeler (2008) use other terms in their definition, including such things as situational or contingency, charismatic, transactional and transformational. Very often the terms used are a reflection of the times the literature was written in and actually have many similarities. I would describe my own leadership style as transformational: by that I believe I endeavour to empower and enable staff and to both manage and lead others towards continued personal and professional development. I see my role as being one of assisting the growth and skills development of individual staff while

(Continued)

(Continued)

also meeting business objectives. This in turn can result in staff being more reflective and transformative in their practice and as a result the cycle continues (Burton, 2006).

There are positive aspects for the mentee and the organisation in engaging in a mentorship relationship, whether this is formal or informal. Aldred et al. (2008) suggest that mentees will benefit through improved performance and productivity, enhanced career opportunities and career advancement. The benefits for mentors are improved performance, greater job satisfaction, loyalty, commitment and an increased self-awareness, resulting in reduced conflict and improved relationships with colleagues and customers. It would seem reasonable to attribute some of the above benefits to managers who mentor. However, the negative impacts may be more pronounced when a line manager mentors. At this level mentoring should be a voluntary exercise which staff undertake, so line managers being mentors may preclude some of the benefits mentioned earlier. Clutterbuck (2008) uses an acronym to sum up what mentors do: **M**anages the relationships, **E**ncourages, **N**urtures, **T**eaches, **O**ffers mutual respect and **R**esponds to the mentee's needs.

Tourigny (2005) suggests well-organised, supported formal mentoring was good for individuals and their organisations; but added that badly organised mentoring was worse than nothing at all. Tourigny (2005) goes on to argue that informal mentoring offers a greater choice of mentor and the direction of development allowing personal preferences rather than those dictated by the organisation. As a manager in the care sector I was interested to read Hafford-Letchfield and Chick (2006) who link mentoring to learning processes that encourage the establishment of learning organisations; they suggest that mentees should be considered as adult learners.

Quinn and Hughes (2007), along with many other writers, have reflected on the work of Malcolm Knowles who compares the ways in which children learn (pedagogy) to the ways adults learn (andragogy). They also discuss the work of Kolb who amongst other things describes different learning styles. It is important to recognise from this work that there are similarities and differences in the way individuals learn and there is some value for mentors in understanding the many definitions of learning styles and the impact a person's learning style may have on the mentoring relationship. Learners will require different approaches to the facilitation of their learning at different points in their learning and careers, dependent on the situation and subject they are exposed to.

As a manager who mentors it is vital to have an awareness of the various theories and styles and recognise where a mentee is in relation to the situation and their potential for personal development. Many writers suggest that learning is cyclic and that part of the process should include reflection: this is a key consideration for mentors. Reflection is seen as important by the GSCC (2002b), and writers such as Lewis (1996), Aldred et al. (2008) and Clutterbuck (2008) suggest that reflection allows the consideration of theory and its interplay with practice.

In conclusion, mentoring is generally perceived as a managed relationship that encourages, nurtures and potentially teaches mentees. The relationship is key, one that is founded on mutual respect and allows sufficient trust and confidence for an open and honest communication in which a mentor is able to respond to a mentee's changing needs. As a line manager my research suggests that it is difficult to provide true mentoring support to those I manage, however, there is symmetry between the roles of mentor, manager and leader regarding the skills required, and I can employ mentoring skills in the existing relationships I have with those I manage to enrich the process of supervision. The potential conflict of needing to take disciplinary action against someone I may mentor adds to the complexity of the relationship. I do think that utilising existing and newly acquired skills within the forum of supervision should add value and inform professional development for those I manage. This in turn will have benefits for the individual, for myself as a line manager and for the organisation, including the recipients of services.

Through my research I have recognised the overlap in the good skills of mentors, managers and leaders and that these are intrinsic to each other. My reading suggests that the advantage of informal mentoring is greater freedom as regards the mentor/mentee relationship and learning and development. Formal mentoring, whilst more limiting in matching mentor to mentee, will have organisational credence with perceived benefits for the organisation and not just the mentee. Good core skills are crucial to effective mentoring; however, these can work in informal settings too, strengthening and widening learners' experiences and opportunities for growth. The knowledge of what motivates learners and when this happens will impact on how I work in the future with my managers to make the most of learning opportunities.

I recognise that the informality of my mentoring approach does make it very difficult to evaluate any changes in practice or assess improvements. Most of my evidence is anecdotal regarding changes in observable behaviours; however, I would note that I have observed more unity together with a greater willingness to be open and honest in mentees' professional discussions. The managers have also become more reflective of their own practice and of those they manage and indeed of the team as a whole.

(Continued)

(Continued)

To summarise, mentoring is best delivered 'offline', if this can be achieved, in order to avoid the disparity of mentoring versus disciplinary roles. Mentoring skills can be effectively employed to enrich supervision and it is important to recognise that adult learners will move between styles that are appropriate to situations and their skills, and also that reflection is valuable in many spheres but particularly in learning. My research has allowed me to consider and evaluate the significance of relationships in learning and how these can be facilitated in practice. Such practice will be different things to different learners at different times so all opportunities should be optimised. I have become acutely aware of the need to better evaluate the learning of those I manage and indeed my own learning.

Chapter link

Consider the impact of your leadership on the relationship with your student. (See Chapter 2 for a further discussion.)

Characteristics for leadership within mentorship

Whatever organisational position mentors are in, they will need a range of characteristics and skills in order to lead practice education effectively. Influencing, motivating and developing others are the important leadership elements within mentorship, not position. Following a review of the literature the following key leadership characteristics emerge as the most relevant: relationships skills, communication skills, motivational skills, role modelling and acting as a change agent. As with mentorship, relationships are the cornerstone of leadership. A leader's ability to establish, maintain and develop relationships is imperative in order to be able to motivate and facilitate others to meet goals or outcomes. This translates to health and social care students in that mentors use their leadership skills to lead and facilitate learning that will enable students to reach their potential along with achieving competencies. Mentors need to demonstrate practice competence and confidence and excellent standards of care delivery to students. George (2003) uses the term 'authentic leadership' to describe a leader whose behaviour is based upon ethical principles and values and high standards of care and having a solid sense of what is important to them both personally and professionally. Schira (2007) describes how authentic leaders are invested in the development of others and work to achieve not only common goals but also the individual goals of those they work with. Mentors should reflect on how they display authentic leadership within their own mentorship role and how they can build on their relationships with students to further enable them to learn.

Chapter link

See Chapter 1 for a further discussion regarding the application of Master's level skills to mentorship.

Both mentorship and leadership are practices that rely on interpersonal interactions, thus excellent communication is imperative for effective leadership within mentorship. Schira (2007) stresses that one of the most crucial skills for an effective leader is being a 'master communicator' who can articulate ideas clearly and openly and share knowledge. Schira's point reflects the assertion of the authors of this book, that mentors need and must therefore have higher level skills in order to fulfil their role. The ability to actively listen is a feature of a good leader's communication style and is important for mentors in relation to their students. Students need to be able to talk to, question and reflect with their mentors about practice and their learning and feel listened to. By listening in a meaningful manner mentors can demonstrate their own enthusiasm for learning from students and others as well as a recognition and commitment to their own development needs.

In professional practice it can be argued that knowledge is power. Watson (2007) suggests that ineffective leaders keep professional opportunities to themselves, do not share and seek personal accolades. Mentors are in a position of power over their students and if they do not openly share knowledge and information with them this will exacerbate power differentials, leading to student alienation and a poor learning experience. The aim of both leaders and mentors is to improve their own practice and that of others, sharing opportunities and valuing those others' achievements. It is therefore vital that mentors share knowledge and information with their students as part of their responsibility to them and their responsibility to develop practice.

Mentors need to display enthusiasm and a passion for caring for patients/ clients and for their profession. Motivation in relation to leadership within mentorship includes skills relating to delegation and risk taking. A key aspect of motivating students is allowing them to progress and maximise their learning opportunities for safely practising their skills. This demands an ability to delegate, which is another feature of good leadership, and requires mentors to facilitate a sense of ability, confidence and accountability in students. Delegation also sometimes requires an element of risk taking; good leaders are able to take risks because they are confident in their skills and knowledge and have earned the trust of others. Students will trust good mentors, thereby allowing the latter to take carefully thought-out risks in order to help students meet their learning objectives. Mentors have a wider remit for facilitating learning in relation to the learning environment and learning organisation: they may consider utilising their leadership skills in relation to taking some risks in order to improve the learning environment. Colleagues and team members will trust a mentor in relation to teaching and learning and see them as a leader for practice education. This allows the mentor to help create a learning environment in which the freedom to express ideas is encouraged and supported, critical thinking is encouraged and others may feel able to take critically appraised risks. An example of this may be a team member undertaking a teaching session for the team for the first time, or the introduction of an evidenced-based innovation that has been effective in a different practice setting but not in the practice area for the team.

Chapter link

The importance of role modelling cannot be over emphasised. (See Chapters 2, 3 and 8.)

Role modelling is a key aspect of being a mentor and mentors should consider how they role model leadership qualities. By leading students practice education mentors are in an ideal position to role model strong effective leadership skills, both in developing professional practice and promoting the profession and by proactively engaging in their own learning as well as that of students. Walker et al. (2011), in their review of leadership characteristics that influence clinical learning, identified that when leaders actively role model knowledge and skills acquisition by teaching and practising in an evidence-based manner, they bring the team together in learning and encourage critical thinking. By being positive, proactive and taking the initiative in practice, a mentor's leadership skills are highly visible to students and this exposes them to the type of leader they aspire to be. Mentors also have a responsibility to nurture and develop students' leadership skills. Mentors for health and social care students need to nurture students so they may recognise their own leadership abilities as well as guiding the development of their own leadership qualities and style. One example here is a mentor highlighting to a student when they have taken the lead on their own learning and encouraging that student to identify appropriate learning opportunities. Given that a degree of leadership ability is required of professionals on qualification, it is vital that students are exposed to mentors who role model leadership appropriately.

The capacity to influence practice, advocate for patients, clients and the profession, and achieve change including managing resistance is integral to leadership. Mentors demonstrate leadership in action to their students by modelling evidence-based practice and critical thinking and engaging with research in order to bring about change. As leaders of practice education, they should regularly review students' experiences based on evaluation and make appropriate changes to the learning environment and planned teaching and learning opportunities. Changes in practice or policy and procedures will involve the team and take time. By contributing, considering and reviewing the learning environment and the learning organisation a mentor can facilitate their own ability to act as a change agent and that of others. Developing and maintaining networks is vital for mentors in securing a wide range of learning experiences for students, particularly when considering the patient/client journey through health and social care services and the current emphasis on hub-and-spoke placements. These established networks with strong communication channels further facilitate the mentor's and the team's capacity for leading change. Part of leadership is being open to learning from others and mentors who encourage mutuality with their students may instigate a change based on learning gained from those students. Vision is a key feature of leadership and mentors can demonstrate their vision by working in partnership with universities contributing their vision of what future practice education should look like.

In the following case study Davison also recognises the shared characteristics of mentors and leaders and considers transformational leadership as an appropriate leadership style for mentors.

Transformational leadership – John Davison

I currently work as a team leader within the Adult Community Nursing Service. I have overall responsibility for six caseloads and I am first line manager for 15 nurses ranging from band 3 to band 6. My area of work is usually a placement for third-year students. Although I have the responsibility now, I have plenty of experience being a 'learner'. I started my career as a Pupil Nurse; I have completed a District Nurse Certificate as an Enrolled Nurse, successfully negotiated the Conversion Course to a Registered General Nurse, and have gained a Specialist Practitioner Qualification as a District Nurse. This has not only reinforced my understanding of what it is like to be a learner throughout my career; it has also given me insight into the differing types and styles of mentors and mentorship. I have also been a mentor both formally and informally for students on a range of programmes, from pre-registration nursing programmes to specialist practice community programmes.

Theories of leadership are not new. Plato referred to 'the Guardians' within ancient Greek society as leaders, commenting that they had a 'higher function' and the ability to lead others to 'enlightenment', or, in the context of nursing, as having more experience and the ability to nurture those who are less knowledgeable, thus enabling their gaining experience.

It is imperative that those mentoring students in the nursing arena have sound leadership skills. Many aspects of good leadership reflect what students see as good mentors. Hyett (2003) comments that leadership should be about encouragement, facilitation and listening, acting as a 'role model' and demonstrating they care for patients and students. Pearcey and Elliot (2004) go further here, stating that we should not only demonstrate caring but also actually care for our students. This is fundamental to our team philosophy: students must not be seen as an inconvenience, but as our future! We must provide information and support, carry out care based on theory and research, have superior communication skills, show concern, and be aware of the needs and objectives of the people in our team. Leaders must act as visionaries who help people plan, lead, control and organise their own activities (Cook, 2001; Mahoney, 2001; Jooste, 2004) and nurses want leaders with drive, enthusiasm and credibility, not just superiority.

Effective mentoring encompasses good working relationships and relevant mentor–mentee communication, including generic and specialist subject expertise and feedback. A good mentor is more than a person who guides and supervises the learning experience and assesses student competencies in the practice area. By empowering students, mentors can enable them to find their own answers and solve their own problems (Wallace and Gravells, 2007). Any nurse educator, a role expected of an effective mentor, must be aware of learning theories to enable the identification of teaching strategies to support learning (Clay and Wade, 2001). Students are encouraged to solve problems using thought processes and reflection; however, mentors must be able to recognise when is the right time to offer help and the level of help that is required. Vygotsky (1978) talks of putting 'scaffolding' in place: this allows mentors to establish the level of support required and adjust that level as students develop. For example, the more a student gains competency in a task the less scaffolding or support they will need to undertake that task. By avoiding pedagogical methods of teaching students can develop their own methods of problem solving, as opposed to being 'spoon fed' and only learning to learn what they are told.

Participative leadership looks at not only being a leader of a team but also at working with and within the team, recognising the different roles and skills of various team members, and including them in decision making. This is also true for mentors. Although a student is assigned to a mentor for the period of their placement, that mentor must use the same characteristics as a leader in order to establish which team member has the knowledge and skills to assist the student in their development in a particular role or task. This style has many similarities with the transformational theory of leadership and in combination seems to be the preferred option for leaders within the NHS. This, it can be argued, is more of a true reflection of leadership as opposed to management, allowing for development, vision, co-operative and collaborative working but not focusing so much on planning, budgeting and goal achievement. It is evident that if people are better developed, both educationally and practically, and are aware of the organisation's vision, the end result will be met but with greater enthusiasm and attention.

Effective mentoring in the health care arena is one of the most important means of developing the leaders of tomorrow. As with leadership theory, mentors will develop through experience, motivation and desire, and must be supported through education and the investment of time to reach their potential. Many of the qualities of a good leader mimic the qualities of a good mentor. Both must be trustworthy, competent and skilled communicators, able to empower the people

(Continued)

(Continued)

who work with them, foster their participation and encourage their sense of being a 'team' in order to facilitate the real development of services. They must also act as a role model for all the people around them, not just learners.

It should be remembered that whatever personal qualities, attributes, knowledge, skills and abilities a mentor has they also have other duties to perform apart from their mentorship role. Students need to appreciate there will be limitations on their time, that they will have a high workload and competing demands between student teaching and patient care (Bennett, 2003). Managers will have their expectations of what they need the health care professional to do, and while they need to support the mentor to enable facilitation of learning, they may also put pressure on the mentor to complete tasks set by them as a priority, thereby leaving that mentor in a very difficult position (Moseley and Davies, 2008). In situations such as this a mentor will need to demonstrate both prioritisation skills and professional assertiveness skills.

It is clear to me that the most effective mentors will be demonstrating the skills, knowledge and values that are also demonstrated by the most effective leaders. It is of paramount importance that mentors are cognisant of role modelling these skills and qualities to learners.

Approaches to leadership

There are many comprehensive books that offer an excellent overview of leadership theories approaches and styles (Barr and Dowding, 2008; Northouse, 2010). In relation to mentorship it appears that as identified by Davison in the above case study, transformational leadership is the style that is of most value for mentors and therefore it will be the focus of the remainder of this chapter. Davison highlighted the need for mentors to care for students as part of their mentor and leadership roles. Schira (2007) suggests that leaders should genuinely care for others and their development. Students have reported the need to feel valued and cared for by their mentors in terms of belongingness. Therefore transformational leadership will be considered in the context of 'caring' and emotional intelligence. While transformational leadership may be the most appropriate approach for mentors to adopt, leaders will utilise aspects of other approaches depending on the situation and context. What follows is an overview of some well-known leadership styles with a potential application to mentorship.

Chapter link

Consider how you enhance student belongingness within the community of practice. (See Chapter 2 for a further discussion.)

Table 9.2 The influence of leadership styles on mentoring approach

Leadership style	How a mentor may use the identified leadership style within mentorship
Autocratic/task orientated	
This form of leadership is when the leader has complete control over colleagues/team members. Team members have no opportunity to contribute to decisions or make suggestions. The approach to activity is task focused, with the leader deciding who does what and how in order to 'get the job done'. Autocratic leaders are focused on output or the achievement of goals as opposed to being interested in the individuals they work with.	A mentor demonstrating an autocratic leadership style will create an extreme power differential between themselves and the student, with the mentor dictating what that student will learn and how. The student's learning will be task focused and may concentrate on the psychomotor aspect of the student's skill base to the detriment of cognitive and affective domains of learning. The mentor will not engage the student in dialogue concerning the student's learning needs and the student will have limited chances to maximise opportunistic learning opportunities. The mentor will focus on the student's documentation and the need to achieve competencies. The student is likely to feel frustrated, unable to contribute and demotivated, and is unlikely to feel valued or reach their potential.
Bureaucratic	
Bureaucratic leaders strictly follow policy, rules and guidance generally without question and expect team members to take the same approach.	A mentor adopting a bureaucratic approach to leadership will encourage the student to learn by following documented policy and guidelines. This may be an appropriate approach in many situations, for example moving and handling or lone worker procedures. However, an emphasis on policy and procedure may limit the student's development regarding tacit knowledge and professional judgement. An over-use of written policy/guidelines may also threaten the student's recognition of patients'/clients' autonomy and the notion of empowerment. In terms of guidance regarding student hours the mentor is likely to adopt a rigid approach, for example not letting a student stay later in order to engage in a learning opportunity.

(Continued)

Table 9.2 (Continued)

Leadership style	How a mentor may use the identified leadership style within mentorship
Laissez-faire Translated, laissez-faire means leave it be. The leader adopting this style believes in the team members being responsible for their own contributions and managing with little input from the leader. This can be a motivating approach if team members are experienced and the leader gives feedback.	A mentor adopting a laissez-faire approach to their student will expect them to plan their own learning to a greater extent. The student may feel motivated and is able to take a flexible approach to learning opportunities and may have a positive learning experience. This experience is further facilitated if the mentor has regular contact with the student to discuss and reflect on learning. The success of this approach will increase if other team members have an active interest in the student. However, many students may feel unsupported and overwhelmed and will need more direction with their learning.
Democratic/people orientated A democratic leader is more focused on the development of individuals as opposed to a focus on tasks. This type of leader encourages team members to participate in the decision-making process, thus improving quality and increasing job satisfaction.	A democratic mentor will involve the student in planning their practice-education experience. While the mentor will make the final decision regarding student competence, the mentor and the student will have regular contact for feedback and reflection. The student will be encouraged to negotiate and participate actively in their learning and is likely to feel valued by the mentor and team and empowered in their learning.
Transformational Transformational leaders are inspirational and successful at motivating others to achieve shared goals. This type of leader is creative and visionary and has considerable influence, encouraging people to move from self-interest to team/organisational interests and goals.	The mentor who has a transformational leadership style will have great enthusiasm for the students learning and development. They will motivate the student to see beyond their immediate goals and consider themselves in the context of the wider organisation. The mentor will have had a positive influence on the learning environment and team members will also be concerned and interested in the student's learning. The student is likely to feel valued and part of the team and experience an excellent learning practice placement. The mentor will need to ensure that the student experiences a balance of achieving immediate goals whilst also considering the wider context.

There are some benefits and limitations to all leadership styles, and in reality mentors will apply the concept of situational leadership when they select the most appropriate style of leadership for a specific situation. That said, transformational leadership appears to be the most popular style within health and social care practice because of its focus on relationships, communication and teams striving together to enact change and meet shared aspirations and goals. It can be argued that transformational leadership has value for mentors in terms of its focus on relationships, open communication and the sharing of knowledge. Northouse (2010) describes transformational leadership as a process involving the leader engaging with individuals and being attentive to the motives and needs of those individuals, thereby helping them to reach their full potential. Wigens (2006) echoes this view, adding that transformational leadership involves ensuring there is feedback on performance, the development of trust and supporting networks, and the use of emotional intelligence. It is clear that many aspects of transformational leadership are crucial for mentors in their relationship with students. Stanley (2008) tempers transformational leadership by suggesting that nurses looking for leadership want less visionary qualities and a greater undertaking of practice activities by leaders that is matched by their values about care and the profession. Stanley describes congruent leaders as still being inspirational, motivating and good communicators, and having a vision for the future, but they are looked to for where they stand now as opposed to where they are going. This approach may have more relevance for mentors who tend to be delivering care in practice as opposed to those who occupy a more senior position with a specifically defined leadership role that may be more suited to transformational approaches to leadership. There are significant similarities between transformational and congruent leadership, one such feature being caring about others, and mentors should consider the balance of their own leadership approach. As identified by Davison in the case study above, good leaders care about their students. In relation to a mentoring programme Snelson et al. (2002) highlighted several key characteristics from caring theory that are of importance both to mentors and mentees. The following aspects are adapted from this work and suggest that caring is:

- an action in which one individual makes provision for another and protects them from difficulties;
- critical to human development and fulfilment;
- a commitment, i.e. the intention to care is a conscious decision;
- a strategy for reducing stress and anxiety and increasing coping in practice.

Students have reported the importance of feeling cared for by their mentors and other team members, identifying excellent mentors as those who offer support, give constructive feedback and broaden student thinking by suggesting alternatives; in addition, they do all of this in a genuinely caring manner. It may be useful for mentors to consider the caring aspects of their relationship and approach to students in the context of emotional intelligence. In relation to nursing, Stickley and Freshwater (2002) suggest that the capacity to care and emotional intelligence will influence the quality of care delivery. Several authors have linked transformational leadership with emotional intelligence (Wigens, 2006; Akerjordet and Severinsson, 2008; Hsu et al., 2011). Emotional intelligence has been defined as an ability to identify, analyse and manage the emotions that will help leaders to cope with demands in a supportive and knowledgeable manner (Akerjordet and Severinsson, 2008). Emotionally intelligent leaders harness their own emotions and those of others when motivating teams. Cummings et al. (2005) assert that nurse leaders inspire by channelling passion and emotions to achieve goals that may not otherwise be revealed and suggest that emotional intelligence is a key factor in transformational leadership. Goleman (1995) identified various elements that define emotional intelligence:

- empathy – the ability to identify and understand the desires, aims and opinions of those around you. People with empathy are good at recognising the feelings of others and are therefore excellent at managing relationships;
- self-awareness – people with high emotional intelligence are very self-aware. They don't let their emotions get out of control because they understand these and are confident in trusting their intuition. They are also honest about their strengths and weaknesses and are therefore able to develop;
- motivation – people with high emotional intelligence are highly motivated and effective. They also enjoy challenges;
- social skills – team players with strong social skills who focus on the success of others. They can manage conflicts, are excellent communicators and are masters at building relationships.

Mentors will recognise many of the above elements as skills that they require to mentor effectively. Northouse's (2010) explanation that emotional intelligence is to do with emotions (affective domain) and thinking (cognitive domain), the interplay between the two and the ability to understand emotions and apply this understanding has resonance for mentors in their quest to facilitate students who are learning in these domains. Following a literature review on emotional intelligence, Akerjordet and Severinsson (2008) found that correlations exist between transformational learning and emotional intelligence, and in particular the possession of empathy. It is evident that there is triangulation between the ability to care, emotional intelligence and a transformational/congruent leadership approach which has significant importance for mentors and mentorship.

Chapter summary

Mentors for health and social care students have a pivotal role in leading the practice education of their students. It is vital that these students are exposed to good leadership and are given opportunities to develop their own leadership skills. This is necessary because when they qualify in their profession they will have to make decisions, act autonomously at times, and strive towards shared team and organisational goals. Through the role modelling of appropriate leadership qualities, including mastery in relationship building and the open sharing of knowledge, mentors can influence not only students' learning but also that of other team members and the learning environment. This influence involves learning becoming rooted in everyday practice. By virtue of their skills mentors have the potential to lead at different levels. These levels are described by Gallagher and Tschudin (2010) as the micro-level, adopting a leadership role with individuals and teams; the meso-level, contributing to organisational debate and policy making; and the macro-level, engaging politically. Mentors may not view themselves as leaders; however, by embracing the challenges of mentorship they will continue to develop their own leadership skills. They should consider their leadership characteristics and approaches in order to increase their capacity for leadership at all levels, and serve their students well by preparing them for the leadership demands of health and social care professional practice.

Reflective activity

After reading the chapter take a little time to consider the activities below:

- What do you look for in a leader?
- How would you describe your leadership style?
- Consider how you role model leadership to students and colleagues.
- Reflect on how you might continue to develop your leadership skills further.

References

Aldred, G., Garvey, B. and Smith, R. (2008) *Mentoring Pocket Book* (2nd edn). Alresford: Management Pocket Books Ltd.

Ali, P.A. and Panther, W. (2008) 'Professional development and the role of mentorship', *Nursing Standard*, 25, 1 (42): 35–39.

Allan, H., Smith, P. and Lorentzon, M. (2008) 'Leadership for learning: a literature study of leadership for learning in clinical practice', *Journal of Nursing Management*, 16 (5): 545–555.

Akerjordet, K. and Severinsson, E. (2008) 'Emotionally intelligent nurse leadership: a literature review study', *Journal of Nursing Management*, 16: 565–557.

Barr, J. and Dowding, L. (2008) *Leadership in Health Care*. London: Sage.

Bennett, C.L. (2003) 'How to be a good mentor', *Nursing Standard*, 17 (36): 1–14.

Burton, J. (2006) 'Transformative learning: the hidden curriculum of adult life', *Work Based Learning in Primary Care*, 4 (1): 1–5

Clay, G. and Wade, M. (2001) 'Mentors or practice educators?', *Community Practitioner*, 74 (6): 213–215.

Clutterbuck, D. (2008) *Everyone Needs a Mentor: Fostering Talent at Work* (4th edn). London: Chartered Institute of Personnel and Development.

Conway, J. (2007) 'The changing skill mix and scope of practice of health care workers in New South Wales: implications of education and training reforms for registered nurses practice, performance and education', *Contemporary Nurse*, 26 (2): 221–224.

Cook, M. (2001) 'The renaissance of clinical leadership', *International Nursing Review*, 48: 38–46.

Cummings, G., Hayduk, L. and Estabrooks, C. (2005) 'Mitigating the impact of hospital restructuring on nurses: the responsibility of emotionally intelligent leadership', *Nursing Research*, 54 (1): 2–12.

Foster-Turner, J. (2006) *Coaching and Mentoring in Health and Social Care: The Essentials of Practice for Professionals and Organisations*. Oxford: Radcliffe.

Gallagher, A. and Tschudin, V. (2010) 'Educating for ethical leadership', *Nurse Education Today*, 30: 224–227.

General Social Care Council (2002a) *Codes of Practice for Social Care Workers and Employers*. London: General Social Care Council.

General Social Care Council (2002b) *Guidance on the Assessment of Practice in the Workplace*. London: General Social Care Council.

George, B. (2003) *Authentic Leadership: Rediscovering the Secrets to Creating Lasting Value*. San Francisco, CA: Jossey-Bass.

Goleman, D. (1995) *Emotional Intelligence*. New York: Bantam.

Hafford-Letchfield, T. and Chick, N. (2006) 'Talking across purposes: the benefits of interagency mentoring scheme for managers working in health and social care setting in the UK', *Work based Learning in Primary Care,* 4:13–24.

Hannagan, T. (1998) 'Leadership'. In T. Hannagan (ed.), *Management: Concepts and Practices* (2nd edn). London: Pitman.

Health and Care Professions Council (2012a) *Standards of Conduct, Performance and Ethics.* London: HCPC.

Health and Care Professions Council (2012b) *Standards of Education and Training.* London: HCPC.

Hsu, H., Lee, L., Fu, C. and Tang, C. (2011) 'Evaluation of a leadership orientation program in Taiwan: preceptorship and leader competencies of the new nurse manager', *Nurse Education Today,* 31: 809–814.

Huckabee, M.J. and Wheeler, D.W. (2008) 'Defining leadership training for Physician Assistant Education', *Journal of Physician Assistant Education,* 119 (1): 24–28.

Hyett, E. (2003) 'What blocks health visitors from taking on a leadership role?', *Journal of Nursing Management,* 11: 229–233.

Jooste, K. (2004) 'Leadership: a new perspective', *Journal of Nursing Management,* 12: 217–223.

Kinnell, D. and Hughes, P. (2010) *Mentoring Nursing and Health Care Students.* London: Sage.

Lewis, G. (1996) *The Mentoring Manager: Strategies for Fostering Talent and Spreading Knowledge.* London: Pitman.

Mahoney, J. (2001) 'Leadership skills for the 21st century', *Journal of Nursing Management,* 9: 269–271.

Moseley, L.G. and Davies, M. (2008) 'What do mentors find difficult?', *Journal of Clinical Nursing,* 17: 1627–1634.

Mullins, L.J. (1990) *Management and Organisational Behaviour* (2nd edn). London: Pitman.

NHS Wales (2010) *Advanced Practice: The Portfolio.* Llanharan: National Leadership and Innovation Agency for Healthcare.

Northouse, P. (2010) *Leadership* (5th edn). London: Sage.

Nursing and Midwifery Council (2008a) *The Code: Standards of Conduct, Performance and Ethics for Nurses and Midwives.* London: NMC.

Nursing and Midwifery Council (2008b) *Standards to Support Learning and Assessment in Practice* (2nd edn). London: NMC.

Nursing and Midwifery Council (2010) *Standards for Pre-registration Nursing Education.* London: NMC.

Pearcey, P.A. and Elliot, B.E. (2004) 'Student impressions of clinical nursing', *Nurse Education Today,* 24 (5): 382–387.

Quinn, F.M. and Hughes, S.J. (2007) *Quinn's Principles and Practice of Nurse Education* (5th edn). Cheltenham: Nelson Thornes.

Schira, M. (2007) 'Leadership: a peak and perk of professional development', *Nephrology Nursing Journal*, 34 (3): 289–294.

Snelson, C., Martsolf, D., Dieckman, B., Anaya, E., Cartechine, K., Miller, B., Roche, M. and Shaffer, J. (2002) 'Caring as a theoretical perspective for a nursing faculty mentoring program', *Nurse Education Today*, 22: 654–660.

Stanley, D. (2008) 'Congruent leadership: values in action', *Journal of Nursing Management*, 16: 519–524.

Stickley, T. and Freshwater, D. (2002) 'The art of loving and the therapeutic relationship', *Nursing Inquiry*, 9 (4): 250–256.

The College of Social Work (2012) *Practice Educator Professional Standards for Social Work*. London: TCSW.

Tourigny, L. (2005) 'A critical examination of formal and informal mentoring among nurses', *The Health Care Manager*, 24 (1): 68–76.

Vance, C. (2002) 'Leader as mentor', *Nursing Leadership Forum*, 7 (2): 83–90.

Vygotsky, L. (1978) *Mind and Society: The Development of Higher Mental Processes*. Cambridge: Cambridge University Press.

Walker, R., Cooke, M., Henderson, A. and Creedy, D. (2011) 'Characteristics of leadership that influence clinical learning: a narrative review', *Nurse Education Today*, 31: 743–756.

Wallace, S. and Gravells, C. (2007) *Mentoring*. Exeter: Learning Matters.

Watson, C. (2007) 'Assessing leadership in nurse practitioner candidates', *Australian Journal of Advanced Nursing*, 26 (1): 67–76.

Wigens, L. (2006) *Optimising Learning Through Practice*. Cheltenham: Nelson Thornes.

Zilembo, M. and Monterosso, L. (2008) 'Nursing students perceptions of desirable leadership qualities in nurse preceptors: a descriptive survey', *Contemporary Nurse*, 27 (2): 194–206.

10 Concluding Thoughts

Case study: Julie Bailey-McHale and Donna Hart

When we first decided to write this book we both believed we appreciated the skill, imagination and commitment required by health and social care professionals to mentor successfully. In the research, discussions and reflections that have taken place over the course of completing this work we have realised how easy it is to underestimate and undervalue the work of mentors. What has struck us time and again is the complexity of the skills, values and knowledge required to do the job well, a job that more often than not is an 'add on' to the already complex professional role of the health and social care practitioner. When we consider that this role is being undertaken within a dynamic practice context that seems forever in a state of flux, then the contribution of mentors becomes even more significant. Pre-qualifying programmes rely on practice mentors to ensure the art, science and craft of the profession is demonstrated in the real world. Without this contribution pre-qualifying programmes could not do what they are designed to do, namely produce competent, committed and inspired new members of the profession. This final chapter will bring together the key themes and learning evident in the preceding chapters, particularly our assertion that mentoring is an advanced activity requiring mastery of both mentorship and professional practice. It will also look forward to the future and what may lie ahead in terms of the role and scope of the mentor in professional practice. We have written our own case study which we hope demonstrates some of the considerations for academics and practice staff when creating a strategic direction for mentorship; it gives some insights into the need for a long-term vision and strategy for mentorship within nursing.

Chapter 1 discussed the qualities associated with Master's level study and made the assertion that these qualities were similar to those required in order to be a skilled mentor. Indeed the premise of this book emphasises that belief. The case studies included within each chapter demonstrate not only the range of knowledge and skills of the mentor writing the case study, but also the application of this knowledge in professional practice and practice education. This scholarly thoughtfulness and dynamic application of theory brings together the key attributes of Master's level practice and this is clearly demonstrated within the domain of effective relationships. In Chapter 2 the range and quantity of the behaviours required to fulfil the characteristics identified by Darling (1984) for effective mentoring is quite staggering, emphasising that successful mentorship is intrinsically linked to the quality of the relationship between a mentor and mentee. It would appear that if this goes wrong the learning experience could be irreconcilably damaged, and indeed some individuals may choose to leave their chosen profession.

One of the key features highlighted throughout the chapters in this book is mentors' need to negotiate quite subtle shifts within the mentoring role. We have seen how the nature of the relationship between a mentor and mentee is crucial, however a mentor also needs to be cognisant of the objectivity required to make an assessment of a student's performance. Indeed in terms of the professional requirements of the role this 'gate-keeping' aspect is extremely important. Chapters 2 and 4 have hopefully given the reader a flavour of the complex skills and attributes demanded in order to do this well. In addition to this, Chapter 5 discussed how mentors must continually evaluate not only the student experience but also their own mentorship skills.

The extensive knowledge base required by mentors has also been a feature of many of the chapters. The range of learning theories associated with the facilitation of learning discussed in Chapter 3 reflects this. The diversity of approaches available to mentors is immense and they are required to select appropriate approaches depending on the individual learner, what is being learnt, the practice setting and the required outcome. Other factors such as a student's learning preference should also be taken into account. One feature of all of the case studies in Chapter 3 is how significant the role of reflection is in learning. In different ways the case study authors demonstrated innovative ways of incorporating meaningful reflective opportunities within their mentoring style.

Many of the chapters have emphasised the importance of the relationship between mentor and mentee; however, another key theme that has significant implications for the mentoring role is the issue of assessment. The potential conflict between the role of mentor and assessor has been debated and it is this divergence in the expectations of the mentor that can make the role so difficult. Arguably, however, it is this role that has the biggest impact on the student, the organisation, the profession and the public. The notion of the mentor as assessor in addition to guide and supporter is a relatively recent add-on, but one that will continue to be a crucial aspect of all pre-qualifying professional programmes. Although there are various examples of professional programmes trying to manage this potential conflict, ultimately a judgement has to be made regarding student competence. An appropriately qualified professional mentor is surely the best person to balance these conflicting roles and ultimately make that decision. Many of the chapters have stressed the increasingly complex nature of contemporary health and social care practice and it is this complexity that makes the task of assessment so difficult.

The following case study details the steps taken within a defined geographical area to construct a considered, collaborative vision of mentorship within that area. It also highlights the benefits of educationalists and service providers working closely in order to secure the best possible preparation for nurse mentors.

Preparing the mentors of the future – Julie Bailey-McHale and Donna Hart

In 2006 the Nursing and Midwifery Council (NMC) introduced new standards for mentorship for all students on NMC-approved programmes. These new standards were subsequently updated in 2008 and have served to concentrate the minds of academics and practice providers alike. This was particularly so as they introduced new responsibilities for practice providers, including the requirement to maintain a live register of mentors, the introduction of sign-off mentors and the setting-up of an appraisal system for mentors, the triennial review. The standards also detailed appropriate preparation for those nurses who wished to be mentors. Most universities had already attached academic credits to mentorship preparation courses, usually at either level five or six. The new standards did not stipulate that mentorship preparation courses should have academic credits, and nor did they stipulate that mentors

(Continued)

CASE STUDY

(Continued)

needed to be educated to a specific academic level in order to support students. However, the changes in health and social care practice and the announcement in 2009 that nursing was to move to all-degree preparation certainly made many nurse academics and placement providers much more aware of their responsibilities within NMC-approved programmes, and especially pre-registration programmes.

In this case study we will describe the journey locally towards constructing a strategic vision for nurse mentorship and demonstrate the absolute necessity of a fully collaborative and committed approach to nurse mentorship by nursing academics and practice leaders. We will also highlight some of the challenges faced along this journey and some of the new challenges arising from contemporary practice, particularly those challenges involved in inter-professional mentorship.

During the academic year of 2005–2006 a review was undertaken locally of the numbers of nursing mentors being prepared. At that time the NMC were consulting over new mentorship standards in the aftermath of work by Duffy (2004) which highlighted the failure by some nursing mentors to fail student nurses who did not meet the required standards. There was much discussion about the academic level of nurse mentors and what was really needed to support nursing students. A review of our local numbers revealed that we had fewer nurses wishing to complete the mentorship preparation module at academic level five. There was also a view within the mentoring team that those who were completing it at level five were doing so because they had high anxieties regarding their academic ability. Many of these nurses successfully completed the level five module with extremely good results. Those who were most successful made the most of the excellent study skills support provided. After much discussion within the mentoring team and with practice leads it was decided that we would only provide mentorship preparation at academic level six. There were some concerns about this decision and a number of colleagues queried whether this would actually deter good nurses from being mentors. As a result the team worked hard at 'selling' the decision to nursing colleagues and emphasised the study skills package available to staff even before they embarked on the module or in addition to the module.

The introduction of the new standards for mentorship (NMC, 2006) produced a surge in the numbers completing our mentorship module; over a two-year period those numbers more than doubled. We had created more work for the team in providing study skills support; however, this work was rewarded with excellent results. Interestingly, when we reviewed figures over a three-year period from the commencement of the move to level six-only preparation, we identified a trend in nurses completing this module and then registering for a full degree programme. It would appear that the successful completion of this module, along with good study support, gave nurses the confidence to go on and complete a full degree.

These excellent results have undoubtedly had tremendous benefits within the practice settings and the support offered to students completing the pre-registration programme. However, both practice leaders and academic staff were keen to capitalise on this success. In 2008 we introduced our first mentorship module at Master's level. We were fortunate to have nursing leaders with the vision and willingness to commit to this venture. Once again, one of the key elements of the introduction of this module was the emphasis on study skills support. We ran an introduction to Master's study workshops in addition to our usual study skills support. Locally, we made the decision to stop delivering the diploma in pre-registration nursing and to only provide an undergraduate programme for nurse preparation from September 2009. This was a key feature of the decision to encourage nurses to access mentor preparation at Master's level. Many were keen to have some experience at an academic level that was above the level of those students they were supporting. We are now in the fortunate position that when our new graduate nurses are ready to access mentorship preparation we will have a strong module ready to deliver at Master's level. Again, this has produced a significant number of nurses who feel ready to embark on a full Master's programme.

There are various new challenges with the introduction of the NMC's (2010) standards for pre-registration education and the move nationally to all-degree-level preparation for nurses. The new standards allow for student nurses to be mentored by other professionals apart from nurses. This move will again require a strategic response and involve practice and education leads across the health and social care community. We think the decisions we have made over the past seven years have placed us in a strong position to respond to these challenges in a constructive and creative manner. We already have a number of health and social care professionals who have accessed the Master's mentorship module and are keen to contribute. The range of other professionals accessing the module includes social workers, physiotherapists and biomedical scientists.

The key to this endeavour has been twofold: firstly, we have ensured that decisions made about mentorship locally have been owned and driven by a collaborative partnership of practice and education leads; secondly, there has been a commitment to be brave about mentorship and to always be one step ahead of the game!

Contemporary health and social care practice is changing. Economic restraints, changes in higher and professional education, and the increased public scrutiny of practitioners have all had an effect on the provision of competent, inspired health and social care professionals. This makes the need for competent and inspired mentors to lead practice education and role model excellence in practice even more vital. We hope this book has demonstrated the advanced skills, knowledge and values utilised by mentors, and that it has shared with the reader a recognition of these attributes as well as a celebration of those mentors who continue to support the next generation of health and social care professionals.

References

Darling, L. (1984) 'What do nurses want in a mentor?', *Journal of Nursing Administration,* October: 42–44.

Duffy, K. (2004) *Failing Students: A Qualitative Study of Factors that Influence the Decisions Regarding Assessment of Students' Competence in Practice.* Glasgow: Caledonian University & Nursing and Midwifery Council.

Nursing and Midwifery Council (2006) *Standards to Support Learning and Assessment in Practice.* London: NMC.

Nursing and Midwifery Council (2008) *Standards to Support Learning and Assessment in Practice* (2nd edn). London: NMC.

Nursing and Midwifery Council (2010. *Standards for Pre-Registration Nursing Education.* Available at http://standards.nmc-uk.org/PreRegNursing/statutory/background/Pages/Introduction.aspx (last accessed 27 March 2012).

Index